How do people come to interpret physical
and psychological changes as 'signs' and
'symptoms' of illness? The aim of this
book is to discuss common under-
standings of health and illness and the
way these may be used to structure our
experience of the world. Three main
approaches have been used in the
attempt to provide a sociological analysis
of illness: Parsons's theory of the sick role,
Mechanic's concept of illness behaviour,
and the explanation of mental illness
offered by labelling theory. Each of these
perspectives has neglected meanings, or
the cognitive and interactional processes
by which meanings are constructed.
Dr Locker argues that meaning is
central to social life. Illness is seen as a
social phenomenon constituted by the
meanings actors employ to make sense of
observed or experienced events.

As a point of departure, contemporary
sociological theory is used to distinguish
between 'disease' and 'illness', and to
demonstrate that there is no necessary
relationship between events in the
biological realm and the social meanings
imputed to them. This position is
elaborated empirically with data derived
from a series of in-depth interviews
carried out with individual women over
the course of a year, and this data is used
to pursue three major issues: (1) the way
in which the respondents were able to
make sense of the problematic
experiences by interpreting them within
a medical frame of reference; (2) the
construction of definitions of illness;
(3) the accounts women gave of how they
managed illness and its associated
problems. A central theme emerging
from the analyses is that events and
situations we face in daily life are always
ambiguous, and it is only through the use
of commonsense knowledge that
meaning and order may be established.

Symptoms and Illness contributes both
detailed and original research data and a
review and evaluation of major writings,
in a fundamental area for discussion and
research in medical sociology.

The author: David Locker is Lecturer in
Sociology at the University of Surrey.

Symptoms and Illness

DAVID LOCKER

Symptoms and Illness

THE COGNITIVE ORGANIZATION OF DISORDER

TAVISTOCK PUBLICATIONS
LONDON AND NEW YORK

B

First published in 1981 by
Tavistock Publications Ltd
11 New Fetter Lane, London EC4P 4EE
Published in the USA by
Tavistock Publications
in association with Methuen, Inc.
733 Third Avenue, New York, NY 10017

Photoset by
Nene Phototypesetters Ltd, Northampton
Printed in Great Britain at the
University Press, Cambridge

British Library Cataloguing in Publication Data

Locker, David
  Symptoms and illness.
  1. Social medicine
  I. Title
  301.5   RA418   80–49716
  ISBN 0–422–77460–X

4/16/82

Contents

*For Geoff
and my Parents*

Acknowledgements

I am especially grateful to David Morgan who supervised the thesis on which this book is based. His consistent encouragement and advice over a number of years and his comments on the early drafts of the manuscript have been invaluable. Many of the ideas presented here benefited from the many discussions we had during the conduct of the research, the analysis of the data, and the writing of the report. Needless to say, he bears no responsibility for the errors, omissions, and inconsistencies that remain. Thanks are also due to Robin Dowie, Christian Heath, and Mildred Blaxter, who commented on the whole or parts of the book. I would also like to thank Dr M and members of his practice for introducing me to some of their patients despite the fact it was unlikely they would benefit in any way from the research. The respondents deserve special mention for the time they gave in answering many questions and the hospitality I received while a guest in their homes. Many others helped, gave support, or kept me amused. Prominent among them were Geoff Posner, Peter Lancaster, Alice Smith, Ruth Watson, Jill Woolford, Paul and Annie Flower, Jill Evans, and Joe Kaufert.

Introduction

Since the 1950s the sociology of illness has been dominated by three main perspectives: Parsons's theory of the sick role, Mechanic's concept of illness behaviour, and the account of mental illness provided by the labelling theorists. To some extent, each of these approaches has neglected meanings or the cognitive and interactional processes by which they are constructed. In this book I argue that illness is a social phenomenon constituted by the meanings actors employ to make sense of observed or experienced events, and explore, by means of detailed case studies, some of the interpretive procedures involved. I also argue that the meanings imputed to these events are important in understanding how they are subsequently managed. Throughout the book I am concerned with the sociological problem posed by illness and illness behaviour and not with the social problem of why people become diseased and why they do and do not use health services.

There are a number of reasons why the issues pursued in this book have been neglected by other writers.[1] Parsons was largely concerned with the production of a comprehensive theory of the social system. His original analysis of illness was designed to illustrate the general process whereby mechanisms of social control operate to reduce the threat that deviance posed to the stability of society (Parsons 1951). The sick role controls the expression of deviant motives in the form of illness by ensuring motivation to recover and resume normal roles.[2] In contrast to Parsons, Mechanic's main preoccupation was with practical problem-solving. His concept of illness behaviour, defined as 'the way in which symptoms may be perceived, evaluated and acted upon by different kinds of persons' (1962:189), is addressed to the problems involved in the effective delivery of medical care. Illness behaviour determines whether diagnosis and treatment will take place, such that systematic differences in illness behaviour in different populations have implications for the need for and provision of medical care.[3] The more radical stance of the labelling theorists aimed to provide a critique of agents and agencies of social control (Pearson 1975). These theorists attempted to show how the labelling and institutional control of the mentally ill created and reinforced the patterns of conduct initially perceived by others as deviant and evidence of illness. Though ostensibly concerned with social meanings, they have been preoccupied with the development and outcome of these deviant careers.

A criticism that can be levelled at each of these approaches is that they treat social phenomena as entities having an existence apart from the consciousness of the actors who engage in or are influenced by them, and/ or see social action being shaped by forces external to and outside the control of the individuals concerned. The alternative position presented here sees social reality as a construct, the outcome of interpretive and definitional work, and social action emerging out of the way in which events and experiences are defined. Some of the propositions of symbolic interactionism and labelling theory are used to demonstrate the centrality of meaning in social life and the writings of Schutz and the ethnomethodologists are used to identify the cognitive processes involved in their production. These are elaborated empirically using case material derived from interviews with six women who were seen several times during the course of one year. The data consists of their accounts of their own experience of health and illness, that of members of their family, and that of others known to them. A major theme emerging from the analysis of this data is that the events and situations we encounter in daily life are always ambiguous and it is only through interpretive work that meaning and order may be established. One of the aims of this book is to describe the way in which the cognitive resources contained within a commonsense understanding of matters of health and illness are used to make sense of experience and provide for the stable, orderly character of the world.

Chapters 1 and 2 provide a theoretical and methodological basis for the analyses pursued in later parts of the book. In the first I attempt to remedy one of the major shortcomings of the sociology of illness by using a particular conception of the nature of social reality to distinguish between those entities referred to as disease and illness. Though often empirically linked, disease and illness are analytically distinct and belong to different realms of experience. I also distinguish between definitions of disorder and definitions of illness and their consequences in everyday life. Because of a general lack of empirical work which could be used to illustrate some of these issues, the limited data available is reinterpreted to show how meanings and actions may be influenced by their immediate social contexts. In the second chapter I outline some of the problems that emerged in the collection and analysis of interview data. Chapter 3 contains some information about the women I interviewed and the persons whose health we discussed. I also provide data to illustrate and justify the view that the accounts they provide in the context of research interviews are constructed in ways such that they may be seen to be moral actors, competent persons, and adequate performers in the social status they occupy. Chapters 4, 5, and 6 are concerned with a detailed analysis of what the women said.

In Chapter 4 I show how the women I interviewed were able to make sense of various events and experiences by interpreting them within a medical frame of reference. These events and situations take the form of cues that disturb the taken-for-granted sense of order and call for interpretive and explanatory activity. A vocabulary of health and illness is but one of a series of alternative ways of organizing and characterizing these states of affairs. Of some importance in organizing these affairs is the context in which they occur. They may be seen in terms of the biography of the individual concerned or related to other events so that meaning and order may be established. I also examine the way in which meaning is given to events in explaining why they occurred or how they came about. Where matters of health and illness are concerned, common sense provides a limited number of theories to account for the past and make the future predictable. One way of demonstrating competence as a member of society is in the use of these socially appropriate explanations in making sense of everyday situations.

While Chapter 4 is about the construction of definitions of disorder, Chapter 5 examines the construction of definitions of illness. I describe the way in which criteria similar to those outlined by Parsons in his discussion of sick-role expectations are used as an interpretive device in lay talk about health and illness. These criteria are employed in the construction of definitions and as prescriptions for action. Here, it is argued that deviance and illness are alternative means of characterizing patterns of action and since definitions of illness involve judgements about responsibility they are essentially moral judgements. Finally, Chapter 6 contains an analysis of the accounts the women gave of the way in which they managed the problematic experiences they encountered. These accounts are treated not as more or less accurate descriptions of what happened, but as reinterpretations of events designed to convey the rationality of their actions. Here, the women are able to show how their conduct *vis-à-vis* consulting the doctor conforms to the criteria which identify responsible patienthood. Any challenge to that conduct by those involved in the delivery of health care constitutes a challenge to their taken-for-granted status as competent persons and moral actors and gives rise to conflict in the patient-practitioner relationship.

Unlike other studies of illness behaviour this book offers no guidelines as to how human conduct may be modified. While other studies have concentrated on the practical problem of individuals who fail to consult in the early stages of serious disease or who consult with 'trivial' disorders, this study is primarily about commonsense knowledge and cognitive processes. This does not mean that it is irrelevant to those involved in the delivery of health care. For the analysis offers one way of understanding how others perceive and·act towards the world. It may be that such understanding is more beneficial than sociological approaches which claim to provide the means whereby human behaviour can be subject to prediction and control.[4]

Notes

1. For a comprehensive critique of the explicit propositions of Parsons's and Mechanic's theories, the institutional contexts in which they were developed, and their infrastructures of sentiment and belief, see Locker (1979).
2. According to this theory, action is the product of internalized roles which are defined by the functional requirements of the social system.
3. The studies generated by this concept have been confined to the identification of socio-demographic and socio-psychological variables which influence help seeking behaviour. Subsequently, models of social action have been constructed from complexes of these variables.
4. For a critique of positivist and interpretive sociologies and their implications for political action see Fay (1973).

1 Labelling theory and illness

In this chapter I present a theoretical appreciation of illness and illness behaviour based on propositions derived from symbolic interactionism and labelling theory. These perspectives are used, not because of any *a priori* definition of illness as deviance, but because their propositions concerning the nature of social reality provide for an understanding of illness as a social phenomenon and their propositions concerning the nature of social action provide for an understanding of illness behaviour.[1] The use of these theories aims to remedy two of the major limitations of the sociology of illness. Beginning with Parsons's definition of illness as 'a state of disturbance in the functioning of the total human individual, including both the state of the organism as a biological system and of his personal and social adjustments . . . It is thus partly biologically and partly socially defined' (Parsons 1951:431), there has been a tendency to confuse disease and illness. Nowhere is this more apparent than in the many discussions of whether illness is a form of deviance.[2] In addition, as I noted in the Introduction, the study of illness behaviour has not taken as its point of departure a theory of social action that accords a significant role to meaning.

Labelling theory

Labelling theory, along with other 'misfit sociologies', was an academic expression of the counter-cultural revolt of the 1960s (Pearson 1975). As such, it offered an approach to the sociology of deviance that was quite distinct from the previously dominant correctional perspective of orthodox criminology. The correctional perspective attempted to identify the causes of deviant behaviour, largely through comparisons of the characteristics of deviant and non-deviant populations, in order to find ways of minimizing the threat it posed to the social order. By contrast, the labelling theorists' commitment was to the so-called deviant and to a critique of those institutions responsible for the control of deviant behaviour. In rejecting the causal approach of the correctional perspective, labelling theory challenged the absolutist view of deviance as an objective entity and focused attention on the social processes which produced deviant outcomes. Prominent among those processes were the activities of agencies of social control.

Labelling theory consists of two types of statements: ontological statements concerning the nature of deviance, and explanatory statements that attempt to account for the development and stabilization of deviant behaviour. The former, essentially an elaboration of the interactionist concept of the social object, are most succinctly expressed by Becker:

> 'social groups create deviance by making the rules whose infraction constitutes deviance, and by applying those rules to particular people and labelling them as outsiders. From this point of view, deviance is not a quality of the act a person commits but rather the consequence of the application by others of rules and sanctions to an "offender". The deviant is one to whom the label has been successfully applied; deviant behaviour is behaviour that people so label.' (Becker 1963:9)

According to Becker, deviance is a community creation. It is not a property inherent in certain forms of behaviour but is conferred on those forms by the audiences that directly or indirectly witness them. It is a social construct, constituted by the imputation of meanings to acts or attributes. Deviance, and social reality, are outcomes of the definitional and interpretive endeavours of participants in social life. The commonsense conception of deviance integral to more traditional sociological approaches 'treats the deviance of an act as existing independently of a community's response. It implicitly posits that certain acts are responded to in particular ways because they are deviant; their deviance is defined by criteria other than the fact that you or I regard or experience the act as deviant' (Pollner 1974). The labelling perspective, however, recognizes that the commonsense actor may believe the deviance to be the cause of his action towards given persons or acts, but sees deviance being constructed by those very actions. Consequently, what does and does not count as deviance is determined in social situations by the actors involved and cannot be defined according to theoretically determined criteria. Sociological definitions of deviance based on norm infraction and rule breaking are inadmissible, for the sociological task is not to define deviance but to investigate the social processes of rule creation and labelling that enter into its production. As Becker notes, while rules and norms create the potential for deviance and are invoked in categorizing acts and actors not all instances of rule breaking become labelled as deviance. Social reaction is highly selective (Linsky 1970; Box 1971).[3]

Labelling theory's conception of deviance has been subject to a number of criticisms, some arising out of the attempt to use this conception in the same way as a normative definition[4] and some the result of misunderstandings which occur because of a loose and imprecise use of terminology by the labelling theorists themselves.[5] As a philosophical assumption, it has not been and cannot be scrutinized empirically. However, the labelling explanation of the development of deviant behaviour has been challenged theoretically and empirically. This explanation relies upon the distinction drawn by Lemert between primary and secondary deviance for the construction of a sequential model of the stabilization of deviant behaviour. Primary deviance refers to rule breaking and is behaviour having 'only marginal implications for the psychic structure of the person concerned' (Lemert 1967:40). Secondary deviance is 'a class of responses which people make to the problems created by the reactions to their primary deviance . . . [it is] deviance committed by people whose life and identity are organised around the facts of deviance' (Lemert 1971:76). The mechanism which transforms primary into secondary deviance is a change of identity and acceptance of a deviant social status on the part of the person concerned brought about by the experience of being labelled, stigmatized, and rejected. In this lies the origin of the tenet 'social control creates deviance'. Many critics of this theory have pointed out that it does not provide an explanation of primary deviance; further, it assumes that the causes of the initial act cease to operate once deviant escalation occurs. Without such an assumption, secondary deviance could be brought about by the continued effects of the causes that produce the initial rule breaking rather than societal reaction and the development of a deviant identity.[6] However, there is a more fundamental objection to this theory, which though sequential, remains causal. That is, there is an unresolvable conflict between the interactionist assumptions upon which the theory rests and its view of the actor as being largely at the mercy of the labelling process. This process determines the actor's identity and future patterns of conduct. As Mankoff points out, these 'implicit notions of human passivity are out of place in a sociological tradition that has been founded on penetrating observations of the creative potential of human beings' (Mankoff 1971:216). This neglect of the actor and his ability to evaluate his own acts and the meanings placed on them by others does not mean that the theory must be rejected but that further theoretical and empirical work is necessary to determine the conditions under which it holds.

Labelling theory and illness

Analyses of illness using the labelling perspective are to be found in the literature though these are largely confined to studies of mental illness. Some of this work is continuous with the critique of the notion of mental illness presented by Szasz (1961) and some applies the idea of a deviant career to mental illness, arguing that labelling and institutional control create and reinforce the sorts of behaviours to which the label was originally applied (Goffman 1968; Wing and Brown 1970). Here, I am solely concerned with labelling theory's ontological propositions and their relevance in developing a sociological understanding of illness, physical and mental. This does not presuppose that either physical or mental illness are deviant states. Indeed, as I will argue later, deviance and illness are mutually exclusive, alternative categories available for explaining and ordering various observed or experienced events.

At first glance the concept of deviance developed by Becker and others might not seem to be applicable to illness. For while deviance may be a property conferred on a person or an act, illness would appear to be an inherent property of a person having a verifiable existence in a biological state which manifests itself in observable or detectable entities called signs and symptoms. Szasz and the radical psychiatrists subscribe to this position when they claim that the disorders we call mental illness are not illnesses at all since they are not the product of demonstrable biological abnormalities. So do more conventional psychiatrists who hold that advances in medical science will eventually lead to the identification of the physiological and biochemical irregularities underlying these problems in living. As Morgan (1975) points out, this implies a view of illness as an objective factual condition of nature, whereby illness is equated with disease and biological and social realms of experience are confused. It is the clarification of this confusion that is sought in the use of the labelling perspective.

According to the labelling approach, deviance is constituted by the meanings imputed by an audience to observable or reportable entities such as acts or attributes. Quite simply, by analogy, illness is nothing more than the imputation of given meanings to similarly observable or reportable entities. Dingwall (1976) has usefully termed these entities 'problematic experiences'. Diseases and illness are then distinct phenomena. Disease is a category applied to a variety of biological events such as changes in physiological, biochemical, or anatomical structure and functioning. As biophysical states these events exist independently of human knowledge and evaluation (Freidson 1970a:223). By contrast, illness is a social state created by human evaluation; it is a symbolic ordering of given events or states of affairs by the application of a label. Consequently, it is not an entity but a meaning used to explain, organize, and evaluate these events or states of affairs.

While the definitions of disease and illness just offered specify the nature of these phenomena they do not encompass the various relationships between them. Disease and illness are not only conceptually distinct, they are often empirically distinct. Someone may suffer from a disease or be subject to some biological abnormality without being defined as ill. Conversely, a definition of illness may be applied in the absence of any medically detectable disorder (Field 1976). Many instances can be found in the anthropological literature to illustrate this point; definitions of illness vary from culture to culture and are independent of disease (Fabrega 1972).

Sociologically speaking, whether or not problematic experiences have a foundation in biology is not essential to their designation as illness. This applies to both mental and physical illness for 'how we apply the label illness is contingent upon the prevailing rationality of social life and not upon the biological character of what is labelled' (Morgan 1975:271). However, it should be noted that when a definition of illness is applied by lay actors it presupposes that an underlying biological disorder is present. In fact, legitimation of the definition of an individual as ill may rest upon the verification of that disorder either by an accepted authority such as a doctor or by the appearance of externally observable manifestations which are independent of the claims of the person concerned.

Although disease and illness are frequently empirically distinct, it is also the case that they are empirically linked. Here, the nature of the underlying biological state and the nature of the manifestations to which it gives rise may have an influence upon whether and when a definition of illness is applied.

I would suggest that problematic experiences, to the extent that they are interpreted in terms of a medical frame of reference, may be symbolically ordered in two ways. First, the individual concerned may define himself or be defined by others as suffering from some biological abnormality. That is, the experiences are interpreted as the signs and symptoms of an underlying disorder. Second, the individual may define himself or be defined by others as ill. There is a qualitative difference between these two states. The latter, while it presupposes the former, involves the allocation of the individual concerned to a social status. This carries implications for that individual's behaviour and relations with others. Thus, the definition of someone as ill has consequences beyond the mere attachment of a label. The former definition, while it may result in that problem-solving conduct called illness behaviour, does not result in a change in a person's social status.

Where problematic experiences are seen to be consistent with a normal order, or seen to have their origins elsewhere, neither definitions of disorder nor illness will be applied. Consequently, problematic ex-periences may or may not have their origins in pathological processes, they may or may not be interpreted as the signs and symptoms of an underlying disorder, and the person concerned may or may not be defined as ill. Labels such as 'signs', 'symptoms', 'disease', and 'illness' are merely one set of resources for organizing and making sense of a variety of observed or experienced events.

The changes in biological and social functioning that may in some circumstances give rise to definitions of illness are, as Morgan indicates, judged against the standards of health and behaviour current in a given society, or its subgroups, at a particular time. Definitions of illness are neither ethically neutral nor value-free. As social constructs, they are moral constructs. Sedgwick (1972) has argued that the category 'disease' is equally a social and moral construct, since it involves man's cognitive organization of nature according to his own self-interests. As he suggests, potato blight consists of a relationship between two living things, a potato and a virus. The designation of this relationship and its consequences reflect man's desire to cultivate potatoes rather than viruses. It is therefore an evaluation of the worth of a given state of affairs. The essential difference is that what is labelled 'disease' has an existence independent of interpretive activity, while illness has not.

On the basis of the above argument, illness is not an entity but a property imputed to a person. As such, it is distinct from disease and illness behaviour. As an explanation of a given state of affairs it may have consequences for behaviour but is not synonymous with that behaviour. Accordingly, I will define illness behaviour as the consequences for social action of the imputation of given definitions to problematic experiences of various kinds. Of course, an individual may do nothing as a result of these definitions; alternatively, he may adopt something akin to what Parsons described as the sick role, or merely indulge in some kind of help-seeking behaviour in an attempt to solve the problem. The theory of social action contained within these statements is derived from the symbolic interactionist conception of the social act (Blumer 1969). That is, it assumes that social action has its basis in the meanings that actors construct to make sense of the events, objects, or states of affairs with which they are confronted. This implies that actors possess the cognitive resources to order the world around them and the material resources to carry out the actions they believe to be appropriate.

The concept of illness career

The concept of 'career' used in sociology has much in common with that used in everyday life. That is, it refers to the progression of an individual through a series of positions in an institution or a social system, each position having implications for the social status of the person concerned. Many authors have conceived of illness as a career and have described unimodal and unidirectional stage models of illness (Suchman 1965; Kasl and Cobb 1966; Kosa and Robertson 1969). By contrast, Freidson employs labelling theory to undertake an analysis of illness as process. He does not apply the concepts of primary and secondary deviance to illness in order to explain how one is transformed into the other as a result of societal reaction; rather, just as diseases pass through identifiable stages, the stages of illness 'are to be observed in human efforts at finding meaning in experience' (Freidson 1970a:240). These are the meanings, imputed by lay actors and agents of social control, that define the illness career.

Fabrega and Manning (1972) employ a similar perspective in their discussion of four types of illness career. These careers are viewed as the product of the medical and social implications of disease and its labelling in medical and lay contexts. The careers are distinguished by the extent to which the disease process is short or long term, curable or incurable, or of sudden or insidious onset, since these determine whether significant modifications in life habit are imposed, relationships with others affected as a result of the meaning the disease holds for them, and whether or not there is significant and long-term change in the evaluation of the person by self and others. Fabrega and Manning would claim that since illness careers may be structured by the labels applied to disease and its consequences, they are not entirely independent of biological reality or of the nature of the problems that are organized by means of these labels. Thus, disease may affect the physical capacity of an individual to behave in certain ways. In addition, the nature of the problems that are experienced may carry different implications for the identity of the person concerned. A short-term acute infection may not involve significant changes in self-identity, it may merely be sedimented into the person's biography, whereas the perceptual and behavioural disorders that come to be called mental illness may bring about a substantial revision of that identity.

The concept of illness career is a useful one in that it identifies and organizes meanings and actions as key components of the social processes that constitute or are the product of illness. However, on the basis of the terminology developed in the previous section, it is limited by definition to those situations in which the label 'illness' is applied. Consequently, it is preferable to speak of a management sequence or episode since problematic experiences which are not ordered by means of such a definition are also managed by a sequence of meanings and actions. Thus, the management sequence begins when some problematic experience is encountered and is the outcome of the social response to multiple phenomena including observed or experienced events, their interpretation in lay and medical contexts, and the socially structured actions taken to cope with these events. The career is neither universal nor unidirectional. Moreover, the meanings and actions by means of which it is constituted are reciprocally related; the imputation of given meanings may have consequences for action which, in turn, may reinforce or bring about a revision in the meanings applied.

Because studies of illness behaviour have concentrated on the socio-demographic or psychological characteristics of users and non-users of medical services, little attention has been paid to the cognitive and interactional processes involved in what I have called a management sequence. Partly because of this methodological bias and partly because of the methodological problems involved, illness behaviour has not been studied as a career. Consequently, there is a shortage of material which can be used to illustrate some of the points made above. Such illustration can only be provided by a reinterpretation of the limited data that are available. Something of the emergent and contextual character of meanings can be discerned in studies by Davis (1963) and Cowie (1976), and something of the emergent and contextual character of actions in studies by Zola (1973) and Robinson (1971).

In Davis's account of fourteen families with a poliomyelitic child, the initial problems reported by the children – sore throats, stomach aches, or fatigue – were often diagnosed as common childhood ailments or interpreted in terms of some prior activity. These ailments were managed by a variety of home remedies. Only one family was alerted to the possibility of polio at this stage since they knew of several other cases in the neighbourhood. In some cases, where the child had a history of malingering, these initial complaints were seen as attempts to gain attention. However, these early diagnoses of the problem were revised when certain events intervened that could not be accommodated within the diagnosis. Davis refers to these as cues. Some were symptomatological, the onset of a stiff neck or the dragging of a leg, and some were behavioural, the inability of a child to win a fight with a younger sibling. In other cases the cue was authoritative: the doctor called in to treat the child's minor illness alerted the parents to the possibility or fact of polio. Cowie describes how the majority of his respondents normalized the onset of chest pain by attributing it to indigestion, injury sustained at work, or the recurrence of a prior illness. The particular diagnosis chosen seemed to depend upon the biographical context in which the pain was experienced. These initial diagnoses were revised and the doctor summoned following a 'critical incident', a sudden increase in the severity of pain, which persisted despite the actions taken to relieve it. The remainder of the respondents quickly realized that they were having a heart attack because of the severity of the pain. It was such that it could not be normalized by reference to previous experience and less serious diagnostic labels.

These studies illustrate something of the process whereby meanings are constructed and support the view that the underlying biological reality may be of relevance in the imputation of definitions. On some occasions the disease may manifest itself in ways which cannot be ignored: it becomes what Schutz (1962) called an imposed relevance. Alternatively, changes in the disease process may bring about changes in subjective experience with the result that the way the problem was originally defined is revised.

By focusing on the timing of the decision to seek care, Zola's study aims to cast light on the observation that only a small proportion of signs and symptoms ever get taken to a doctor. Using interviews with patients, many of whom had tolerated their symptoms for fairly long periods, who were attending a hospital clinic for the first time, he described five non-physiological triggers to the seeking of medical care, such as the occurrence of an interpersonal crisis, sanctioning on the part of others, and interference with physical or social activity. These triggers caused the patients' accommodation to the symptoms to break down and stimulated the seeking of medical aid. While Zola does not offer a theory of social action to indicate how the triggers operate to stimulate help-seeking, his results can be interpreted in terms of the framework offered above. Thus, the 'clinical iceberg' is the product of differences in the way problematic experiences are defined and managed. A given problem may be defined as a disorder worthy of medical attention in one context, but not in another. The triggers Zola has identified are situational factors taken into account when the meaning of events is being constructed, such that the advent of a trigger leads to a change in the way a problem is defined and a change in the action taken to deal with it. Though Zola's study has been criticized on methodological grounds, it does provide for a view of meanings and actions as emergent and context-bound.

Robinson also provides data that illustrate the situational construction of meanings and actions. He quotes the case of Mrs M who, in an interview after her husband has suffered a knee injury, attempts to assess the problem in the light of Mr M's current life situation:

(Mrs M) 'It wasn't too bad when he came in, just tender round the knee. It was stiff Sunday and I said he'd have to go to the surgery Monday . . . but he wouldn't. He started his new job with X's and you can't go sick on the first day. He'd have got his note no trouble last month. Last week he was home anyway (between jobs) and I could have looked after him. Just rest and he wouldn't have needed the doctor. Trust him to do it when he can't be on the sick. Next week he can make out he did it on the site. It's not that bad, mind.' (Robinson 1971:14)

Mrs M has certain notions about when it is appropriate for Mr M to be on 'the sick'. These notions and the context of his work situation influence the definition applied to Mr M's problem and the choice of a course of action. Different contexts are anticipated as giving rise to different interpretations and actions. 'Last month' when Mr M was with his old employer he could have 'gone sick' after getting a note from the doctor. 'Last week' when he was at home between jobs he could have defined himself as sick and acted accordingly without recourse to medical approval. 'This week', however, Mr M had started a new job and because it would create a bad impression to have gone sick on the first day, he had not been able to stay at home and rest the knee.

The situational construction of meaning

So far, I have attempted to clarify illness and illness behaviour by means of a theory of social reality and a theory of social action. Central to both are the construction of meanings. I have used the work of others to argue that two possible influences on the process of meaning and action are the nature of the problematic experiences with which an individual is faced and the nature of the situation within which they occur. How these two concerns may contribute to that process has not yet been fully described. What is now required is a more detailed theory of meaning. This demands an analysis of the way the world is cognitively organized and an understanding of the interactional context in which it takes place.

It is at this point that labelling theory ceases to be directly useful for, as Douglas (1971a:142) has indicated, it is deficient on both of the above counts. It either treats the process of meaning construction as non-problematic and does not explore the process that leads individuals and acts to be assigned to categories or, as I have shown, it has been guilty of an 'asymmetric bias' in which meanings are imposed on the actor by those around him. Consequently, the analysis will be extended using the work of Schutz and the ethnomethodologists. To the extent that they describe the cognitive tools via which social reality is constituted, they provide the basis for a theory of meaning.

Schutz's sociology of commonsense knowledge is focused upon the world of everyday life, the world which is both the scene and the object of our actions and interactions.[7] This world is seen from within what Schutz calls the natural attitude; it is taken for granted as a world of well circumscribed objects with definite qualities, which is known and shared by others. Man's interest in this world is largely practical, he is concerned with doing and achieving and not with acquiring a coherent understanding of the way in which it works. Rather, knowledge of the world is organized in terms of degrees of relevance to his actions and is only as systematic as it need be for the realization of his practical projects. This knowledge of the world and the biographical experiences from which it is derived provide the means whereby new experience may be interpreted. Given that every individual finds himself in a unique, biographically determined situation with a unique stock of knowledge at hand, Schutz is concerned to explain how members of a group come to hold a common view of the world despite their individual perspectives. The solution to this problem is important in understanding how social order is both given in the form of culturally prescribed meanings and also created by individuals in their everyday interpretive activities.

According to Schutz, a common conception of the world is generated by the interpretation of unique experience in terms of a shared sense of social structure. This is facilitated by a process of selective attention that Schutz calls typification, which reduces the unique to the general. This involves the sorting of phenomena into a limited number of classes so that their attributes are equalized and their differences disregarded. Commonsense knowledge consists of a multitude of such types, and once an object has been identified as a member of a given class, characteristics may be imputed to it that are not directly perceived. The world appears stable and orderly to the extent to which events and phenomena are seen to be instances of these types. Language is important in this process, since the language of everyday life is primarily a collection of named things and every name includes a typification. Not only does typification provide for the cognitive ordering of the world, it is also a prerequisite for interaction. Successful interaction can only proceed given mutual understanding. This in turn depends upon congruence between the typifications used by the actor as a scheme of orientation and those used by his fellow men as a scheme of interpretation. Mutual understanding is also promoted, and interaction facilitated, by two idealizations or assumptions. These are the idealization of 'the inter-changeability of standpoints' and that of 'the congruency of the systems of relevance'. Accordingly, I accept

> 'that the differences in perspectives originating in our unique bio-graphical situations are irrelevant for the purposes at hand of either and that he and I assume that both of us have selected and interpreted the actually or potentially common objects and their features in an empirically identical manner, that is, one sufficient for all practical purposes.' (Wagner 1970:76)

The system of typifications, learned and acquired through experience, is organized into a series of recipes. These are culturally or personally prescribed sequences of typifications involving typical problems, typical solutions, and typical actors. They are used both as a precept for action, whoever wants to bring about a given end has to proceed as indicated, and as a scheme of interpretation, whoever proceeds by a given recipe is taken to intend the associated result. Thus, a recipe transforms 'unique individual actions of unique human beings into typical functions of typical social roles originating in typical motives aimed at bringing about typical ends' (Wagner 1970:52). In this way, action is rendered meaningful.

Schutz is primarily concerned with the structure, as opposed to the content, of commonsense knowledge and how such knowledge provides an actor with a scheme for interpreting the natural and social worlds. His work has been extended by the ethnomethodologists in several ways.

First, they have demonstrated empirically that the idealizations or 'background expectancies' Schutz describes are an integral feature of the commonsense world and that interaction cannot proceed if they are breached (Garfinkel 1967). Second, they have begun to identify and to describe the interpretive procedures integral to commonsense reasoning and the labelling process. Cicourel (1973) calls these 'basic rules' and sees them as invariant properties of everyday practical decision-making whereby sense is assigned to an environment of objects.

The focus of Garfinkel's work is the methods by means of which members of a society 'produce and sustain the sense that they act in a shared, orderly world in which actions are concerted in stable, repetitive ways' (Wilson 1971:28). The most fundamental of these is the documentary method of interpretation whereby meaning is given to an observation by seeing it as a surface appearance pointing to an underlying pattern. These surface appearances both point to and are elaborated by that pattern, while the pattern is in part constituted by those appearances. McHugh (1968) used experimental situations to specify the dimensions of emergence and relativity which allowed participants to make sense of random and contradictory responses to their remarks. The subjects assumed that there was some meaning to what was being said and having made a tentative definition of what was going on used subsequent occurrences to elaborate, substantiate, or revise the initial theme. When particular statements were radically at odds with the initial definition imputed, that definition was seen to be a misinterpretation or it was assumed that future events would clarify the discrepancy so as to maintain the original definition. In some cases, however, the interpretive procedures available did not allow these discrepancies to be resolved and led the subjects to question the status of the experiment itself. In this way meaning was given to the fact that an underlying pattern of meaning could not be located.

Because an individual's stock of knowledge is inconsistent and incomplete, meaning construction is always potentially problematic. While some experiences may be readily and unequivocably interpretable, many give rise to a situation of doubt in which their significance cannot be determined. As Wagner puts it:

'External phenomena which come to the attention of an individual may be experienced in ambiguous forms. Thus, doubtful situations arise for the individual, situations apparently containing mutually exclusive tendencies, each of them equally plausible. As a consequence, if a person faces such an ambiguous situation, he will oscillate between possibilities and counter-possibilities. His indecision will last until he finds additional evidence in favour of one or the other alternative or else his own interests or motivations push him in one direction or another.' (1970:29)

As I will show in later chapters, where the interpretive scheme available is insufficient to make sense of or identify a given object, then its context may be invoked and may furnish the grounds for imputing status and significance. In some cases, however, doubt remains and the definitions that are constructed are not employed with any degree of certainty.

Meaning construction is also problematic because it does not take place within a vacuum but within 'actual and potential interaction with others' (Douglas 1971a:203). Consequently, meanings must be acceptable to or may be challenged by co-interactants. All instances of labelling may require justification in terms of the consistency between the characteristics implied by the label and the characteristics of the item so labelled. This is particularly the case with deviance in which one label may supplant another higher up in the moral hierarchy. This 'recasting of the objective character of the perceived other' (Garfinkel 1956:421) may call for a demonstration of the fit between the label and all it implies and what is otherwise known about the individual. This consistency may be achieved by biographical reconstruction. The past is reinterpreted so that acts, events, and objects formerly interpreted as something else come to be seen as indicative of what is now known. It is in this way that meanings are negotiated by the parties to interaction.

The central tenet of the perspective I have elaborated is that an understanding of social life and its constituent phenomena must be derived from a theory of meaning. Social reality and social action are constituted by and emerge out of the meanings that actors construct as they attempt to make sense of and manage the experiences they encounter in everyday life. Consequently, one task for sociology is the documentation of the meanings employed in rendering experience sensible and manageable and the analysis of the processes by means of which the definitions involved are constructed. Manning, talking specifically about the sociological study of organizations, describes the issues to be pursued in empirical research in the following way:

'How [the actor manages the problems that face him] is seen in the devices he uses to make them consistent, repetitive, normal and natural. By means of his linguistic behaviours the actor selects things which through naming become social objects. That is, they have a potential for action when they are named, counted, assessed and ordered. The fashioning of order takes place as objects at hand become named as part, in the context of, or standing for, order. The primary rule for the study of organisations from a phenomenological point of view is that one must study the ways in which terms of discourse are assigned to real objects and events by normally competent persons in ordinary situations.' (Manning 1971:244)

This specification of the topics that require empirical clarification means that the ensuing analysis is directed towards a description of the way in which events and phenomena are assigned to categories. This is the central aspect of the process that results in the imputation of meaning and the construction of social order. As Phillipson expresses it, 'the constitution of socially meaningful realities, achieved largely through language, becomes a basic issue for investigation' (Filmer *et al.* 1972:81). As far as the sociology of illness is concerned, Freidson has outlined some of the issues which need to be investigated:

> 'The problem is to manage the idea of illness itself – how signs and symptoms get to be labelled or diagnosed as an illness in the first place, how an individual gets to be labelled sick and how social behaviour is moulded by the process of diagnosis and treatment.' (1970a:212)

Some of these issues are pursued in later chapters using respondents' accounts of how they managed, cognitively and practically, the problematic experiences with which they were presented. In the chapter that immediately follows, I outline some of the problems that emerged in the collection and analysis of those accounts.

Notes

1. Where labelling theory has been used in an attempt to understand illness, it has been based on a view of illness as a form of deviance. See Freidson (1970) and Dingwall (1976). This basically Parsonian position has been the subject of a protracted if muted debate.
2. See, for example, Butler (1970), Robinson (1971), and Pflanz and Rhode (1970).
3. This forms the basis of the sociological critique of officially collected statistics. As the product of the activities of agencies of social control they do not document the 'real' incidence of rule-breaking behaviour.
4. See the critique of the labelling perspective by Gibbs (1966).
5. It is often claimed that Becker's typology of deviance, particularly his categories 'secret deviance' and 'falsely accused', imply normative conceptions of deviance. In fact, these terms refer to a relationship between rule-breaking behaviour and deviance. Consequently, the events to which they refer are consistent with the labelling perspective; the confusion arises because of an unfortunate use of terminology. For elaboration of this point see Locker (1979).
6. For a discussion of this assumption of aetiological discontinuity see Taylor, Walton, and Young (1973:151–3).
7. This discussion of Schutz's sociology of commonsense knowledge relies heavily on Wagner's (1970) edited volume of his writings from which all quotes are taken.

2 Method and theory of method

Many of the recent critiques of positivistic, conventional, or absolutist sociology have been developed from within a naturalist perspective. On the basis of a commitment to meanings and the view that social life is a product of cognitive and interactive processes, symbolic interactionism, labelling theory, and ethnomethodology have claimed that positivism and absolutism not only mistake the character of the social world but distort that world in the application of a natural science methodology. Positivism is not simply a set of methods which may be used to study the social world, it is a paradigm and involves assumptions about the nature of man and social phenomena. By contrast, naturalism is not a set of methods but a philosophy of method. Integral to this philosophy is some notion of a relationship between the phenomena under investigation and the methods by which they are studied. The naturalist critique of positivism is not then a debate about methods as such but a debate about the appropriateness of certain methods for the study of man and society. Methods are appropriate or inappropriate to the extent to which they retain the integrity of the phenomena to which they are applied. Consequently, under the auspices of naturalism, questions concerning the nature of the events to be studied underlie all methodological disputes.

The view that the social world is inherently meaningful and social reality a construct of the participants within it implies a great deal about what topics are available for sociological investigation and the way in which they should be approached. Research techniques derived from the natural sciences are to be rejected because they do not provide access to these topics and because they objectify social reality, treating man as if he were determined by forces outside of his control. All varieties of sociological naturalism place some emphasis on the categories actors employ to structure their experience of the world and make sense of their social and physical environment. These categories take the place of the concepts sociologists employ in their attempts to explain social reality. This emphasis on the subject's own categories and the methods he uses to create order does not mean that sociology's task is solely one of describing the subjective world as it appears to the participants. Rather, the aim is to move beyond individual experience to reveal the shared assumptions about social life and the activities associated with them which generate and sustain such experiences (Filmer *et al*. 1972).

These concerns determine the way in which the study of social life is to be approached, for as Blumer has said with regard to the study of social action:

'The premise that social action is built up through a process of noting, interpreting and assessing things and of mapping out a prospective line of action implies a great deal as to how social action should be studied. Basically put, it means that in order to treat and analyse social action one has to observe the process by which it is constructed. . . . The required approach is to see the acting unit confronted with an operating situation that it has to handle. . . . This means seeing the action as it is seen by the actor, observing what the actor takes into account, observing how he interprets what he takes into account, and seeking to follow the interpretation that led to the selection and execution of one of these pre-figured acts.' (1969:56)

Blumer's recommendation to observe the construction of social reality frequently involves communication with the members of a society or a group. Douglas considers this the only way of getting at social meanings (Douglas 1971b:9). Communication with the subjects of sociological research may be direct or indirect. Indirect communication occurs via the medium of structured questionnaires. These provide the respondent with a set of preformed categories to be used to describe, and into which he must fit, his experiences. At best, this distorts that experience by the imposition of a structure; at worst, the data produced bears no relation to the subject's experience and merely represents his attempts to accomplish the task of respondent by providing answers to the interviewer's questions. By contrast, what I have termed direct communication allows the respondent to describe his experience in his own terms, it gives access to his categories and the way in which they are used in the production of a cognitive order. Garfinkel (1967) refers to these descriptions as accounts. These accounts may be collected by recording naturally occurring talk, that is, conversations which take place between participants in everyday interaction, or by the open-ended interviewing of informant-respondents. The latter are individuals who participate in or observe the settings or events under study which may or may not be open to participation or observation by a researcher (McCall and Simmons 1969).

Decisions determining the research strategy

Doing sociological research involves managing a variety of theoretical, practical, and methodological problems. In Chapter 1, I outlined a theoretical approach to the problem posed by illness and illness behaviour and identified issues to be clarified and developed by empirical research. The practical problems I faced largely revolved around the choice of a setting in which to pursue these issues and how to gain access to them, and the methodological problems concerned the techniques to be employed to collect and analyse relevant data. In many ways these problems are interrelated; the theoretical perspectives I used had an influence on the techniques by means of which I gathered data, as did the particular settings in which I chose to explore the topics indicated by the initial theoretical work. In turn the data gathering techniques had an influence on the nature and status of the data I had at my disposal and the way in which it could be analysed sociologically.

Because I was interested in the lay construction of definitions of problematic experience I assumed that the family, rather than the doctor's surgery, the outpatient clinic, or the hospital ward was an appropriate setting to study since an important part of the interpretive work involved would take place within the context of family interaction. Of course, such definitional activity may and does occur within a variety of other interactional contexts such as work, recreational activity or contacts with friends, strangers, or medical personnel. From a purely practical point of view the family is a convenient setting to study since it is more easily identifiable and accessible than these alternative contexts.

In many cases, and perhaps fortunately so, the research strategies available to a researcher are limited by the kinds of situations being studied. For example, the types of activities that constitute the setting, and the structure of the interaction within the setting, may determine whether overt or covert approaches are possible.[1] In this study it seemed self-evident that a covert approach was not feasible given the absence of any legitimate means of gaining access to family units for periods of time long enough to collect the necessary data. Since membership of the family is determined by marriage, descent, or adoption it is not possible for an observer to pass as a member. Nor are there any viable roles that can be occupied in order to gain access to the setting. Similarly, the nature of the research situation also determines which methods of data collection may be used. Owing to the particular nature of the family, I decided that access to the setting was too restricted to allow the long-term participation required to observe the interpretation and management of problematic experiences within family interaction. Like Voysey (1975), I assumed that it would be difficult to find families willing and able to tolerate the presence of a stranger in their home, and that the research could not be undertaken without considerable disruption of family activities. It also seemed to me to involve a considerable waste of time; after all, coping with illness is only a small part of family activity. When it was pointed out to me that some had undertaken participant observation of family life my motives became clear; like others faced with the same decision 'I was not prepared to commit myself that much to the project, I preferred to stay at home' (Voysey 1975:75).

Because of the difficulty of bringing off true participant observation, intensive interviewing was employed as the main data-gathering technique. This means that I was limited to obtaining informants' accounts of problematic experiences, their cognitive organization, and practical management. Information was collected in two ways: tape-recorded semi-structured interviews, and health diaries kept by the informants. I decided to use women as informants and interviewed the mother of the family since I assumed that she would be closely acquainted with the problems I wished to discuss and would be more likely than any other individual to be willing to spend time talking about them.[2]

Making contact

The family settings that I wished to study I conceived of as 'ordinary' families. That is, I did not require them to be any more extraordinary than to consist of one or more adults and one or more children. I had some idea that there would be some variation in the matters I wanted to investigate according to such factors as sex and age so that when I had to stipulate the sort of families in which I was interested I asked for one adult of each sex and at least two children. It could be argued that the family settings to which I gained access were far from ordinary, but they are families just the same. At the outset I did not require that the families were special in any way but nor did the fact that they might be said to be special lead me to exclude them from the study.

Though 'ordinary' families are everywhere, there is a sense in which they are nowhere. That is, their ordinariness did not mean they were easy to locate. Other than knocking on doors at random there are no immediately obvious ways of contacting families. Like Bott (1971), I eventually employed the referral method and contacted subjects through an intermediary known to us both. Two women were contacted via acquaintances to take part in a pilot study and the women in the main study were contacted via their GP. I was introduced to a GP who agreed to make an approach to respondents whose families fulfilled the research criteria. He supplied me with a list of five women who had agreed to be interviewed and these were contacted by telephone and letter. I told them that I was interested in the kind of health problems they encountered and how they coped with them.

Unlike quantitative methodologies, qualitative approaches have no equivalent of the statistical and sampling theory to determine matters such as the number of individuals to study. A search of the literature suggested that twenty to fifty interviews is a standard case-load, though this may vary according to the support facilities available. As a PhD student with nothing but a tape recorder and a box of tapes I aimed to conduct thirty interviews since this seemed about the number I could comfortably transcribe and analyse. Since I wanted to interview each respondent several times, the number had of necessity to be small. My original intention was to interview two groups of five women over periods of six months. At the end of the first six months' interviewing I revised this intention and continued to interview the same women for a further six months to take advantage of the relationship that had developed. I also continued to interview one of the pilot cases and subsequently analysed that along with the data I obtained from the five. This seemed justified given the quality of the data that I was collecting. Over time the women had become accomplished respondents; they were able to provide long and detailed descriptions of their everyday affairs and much of what they said was spontaneous.

I did not conceive of the women I interviewed as 'cases'; they are not the unit of analysis. Nor are the thirty or so individuals about whom the women talked. The unit of analysis is what I have referred to as a management sequence. Consequently, interviewing only six women did not reduce the number of units to which I had access. As with any qualitative study that does not investigate a large sample from a defined population, it might be said that the results reported in later chapters are not generalizable and that what I have described is nothing more than the experiences of six women. However, since my intention was to identify some of the constituents of the stock of knowledge available to members of our culture to organize and make sense of their experience, it could be argued that the commonsense understandings the respondents used as a resource in constructing both their accounts and social reality are common by definition and do not have to be shown to be so by large and/ or representative samples of women. This does not mean to say that the frame of reference described is employed universally, merely that it constitutes a resource that may be drawn on for making sense and assigning meaning.

Collecting data

Data was collected by means of tape-recorded interviews, some of which were based on health diaries kept by the respondents. The interviews were conducted in the respondents' homes between May 1974 and June 1975. I preferred to interview the respondents alone, though the husband of one respondent was present at one of the interviews and at interviews with two others the children were sometimes present. At the first interview I asked the respondents if they minded the conversation being taped, explaining that it made recording of what was said much easier for me. At the second interview I mentioned the tape recorder again but at subsequent interviews I took the matter for granted. None of the respondents objected to, or seemed worried by, the use of the tape recorder. The first interview was based on a common schedule designed to encourage the women to talk in general terms about health and illness and to provide details of their family's medical history. I also asked for details of problems that had been experienced more recently, how they had arisen and how they had been dealt with. At subsequent interviews I followed up what had been said in previous interviews and collected information on problems which had been encountered in the intervening period. The respondents were interviewed between three and six times, the difference reflecting the ease with which the women could fit me into their busy daily routines.

I attempted to make the interviews as much like a conversation as possible. Consequently, the schedule I employed was brief. Apart from the initial interview where I collected background information, it con-sisted of a list of individuals the women had talked about, a list of the problems they had discussed, and a set of questions intended to obtain a full account of what was happening or had happened to those individuals and those problems. At each interview these individuals and problems were discussed in turn and I asked, 'What happened?' 'When did it happen?' 'What did you think it was?' 'Why that?' 'What did you do?' 'Why that and with what result?' It was often unnecessary to ask the respondents these questions; much of the information I sought was contained in the lengthy accounts they gave. I used these sorts of questions not only to obtain information on specified topics but also as devices to stimulate the women to continue to talk.[3] In fact, the questions I asked frequently went unanswered although they did bring forth more detailed and elaborate descriptions of the issues under discussion.

Prior to two of the interviews, I asked the respondents to keep health diaries. These were simple records of symptom experiences and actions taken and though they were originally intended as data collection devices I used them only as aids to interviewing. They were sent to the respondents through the post, kept over a period of two weeks, returned to me through the post and formed the basis of an interview which was conducted as soon as possible after the diary was completed. I used them in an attempt to build on the work of Robinson (1971) and others although I wished to avoid their manifest tendency to impose a structure upon the respondents' experiences. As it turned out the diaries were inadequate as sources of data simply because they did not contain sufficient detail. However, they were successful as devices to facilitate recall and provided a systematic record of events which I used in formulating questions and probes. In fact, the difficulty of remembering the exact sequence and timing of events led one respondent to suggest that she keep a diary before I had a chance to suggest it myself.

Though some of the interviews used diaries as a guide they were not in fact constrained by them, and I attempted to clarify the status of the events recorded in the diaries in terms of the respondents' own categories and also to locate instances of events which were not recorded in the diaries since they were not seen by the respondents as falling within the categories the diary demanded. What the respondents said at interview was then used as data and not what they had written in their diaries.

Overall, I conducted twenty-six interviews each of which lasted from three-quarters of an hour to two hours. One of the interviews was accidentally taped over, one was lost due to a fault in the tape recorder, and another disappeared when the tape recorder and the tape it contained was stolen. The remaining twenty-three interviews furnished approximately forty hours of taped conversation which was transcribed in full. Fragments are reproduced in Chapters 3 to 6 with the minimum of editing, although they have been punctuated to avoid the elaborate systems of notation required to make everyday conversation readable.

During the time I conducted the interviewing the respondents seemed unsure of my status. Though I presented myself as an independent researcher, for part of the time at least they seemed to think that I was in some way connected with their doctor's practice or a representative of some other authority. While I wished to preserve my legitimacy by maintaining some link with the practice, I wanted to avoid being too closely identified with it in case complaints and criticisms were inhibited. In addition, two of them found it difficult to accept that I was interested in what they had to say about their 'ordinary' problems and sometimes felt that they had not been very helpful. Consequently, I had to convince them that they were helping me and took to pointing out that I would not have returned to interview them further if what they had to say was of no value.

The analysis of respondent talk

The way in which respondents' accounts of events may be analysed sociologically depends upon the kinds of assumptions one makes about the nature of those events and the nature of the techniques used to study them. The former involves a theory of social reality and the latter a theory of research activity.

Garfinkel has drawn a useful distinction between correspondence and congruence theories of social reality.[4] The correspondence theory seeks to maintain a distinction between the subjectively perceived object and the concrete object such that an analysis may distinguish what 'appears' to be the case and what actually is. From this point of view respondents' accounts are to be treated as more or less accurate descriptions of the events being studied and are sociologically useful only in so far as they are valid. If they are taken to be valid then they may be used to construct or confirm theories about those events. By contrast, the congruence theory proposes that the perceived object is the concrete object and that there is no distinction to be drawn between them. Accordingly, accounts given by respondents are not more or less descriptions of past or present events but merely one account of events that have been accounted prior to the interview and will, doubtless, be accounted again in the future. The interview produces one account out of 'indefinite elaborations of the same scene' (Cicourel 1973:111) each of which may produce different outputs, such that the way in which an event is reconstructed in the context of an interview may not resemble the way it is reconstructed on other occasions. All of these accounts are of equal validity, for none can be judged against an independent reality to see how far it is true. Rather, reality is reconstructed anew in each of these individual accounts. Consequently, the aim is not to use these accounts to determine the viability of a theory about an objective order, since that order is produced in the process of formulating an account. The aim is to use respondents' descriptions of events in order to identify the interpretive and comprehension processes via which social reality is constituted. While a positivistic approach is consistent with a correspondence theory of social reality, symbolic interactionism and ethnomethodology are consistent with this congruence theory.

Both of these perspectives on social reality are associated with distinctive views concerning the nature of the research act. As Phillipson (Filmer *et al.* 1972) points out, the conventional view is that research procedures are neutral devices for providing data to support or falsify theoretical ideas. That is, they provide access to an underlying order that is not otherwise observable.[5] They are taken to be problematic only to the extent that a research design or its execution may induce bias and threaten the validity of the patterns revealed. A more phenomenologically oriented sociology would hold that because the social world is not objective but objectified social order is created rather than revealed by the research process. That is, what are treated as data are not collected during the course of the research act but are a product of that act. As such it is a situational construct.

Phillipson (1972) has argued that in order to collect data a researcher must form minimally meaningful relationships with others and that the data from such relationships emerge out of a process of mutual interpretation. Similarly, Cicourel (1964) has argued that field research is negotiated in much the same way as routine social interaction, such that the meanings produced in the context of the interview are integral to the way in which the subject manages the encounter. Simply put, 'statements by the [respondents] are behaviour towards the investigator in the research situation' (Voysey 1975:73). In fact, the interaction can only proceed given the ability of both participants to make sense of each other and recognize the meaning in what is said. In this way, every field study provides the opportunity to develop theory on face-to-face interaction as well as on substantive topics.

So far I have advanced two claims. First, that accounts given by respondents in the context of the interview are to be treated as phenomena in their own right and not as representations of objective events or states of affairs. Secondly, that these accounts emerge out of a particular social encounter. Consequently, in analysing what the respondents said, I have assumed that the interview provided them with one opportunity for constructing and reconstructing the meaning of their experiences and that these meanings were selected according to their purposes in participating in the interview. That is, I take their accounts to be constructed in ways which allow them to be seen as moral persons, competent members and adequate performers in particular social statuses and their experiences seen to be consistent with a known and routine order of things. It is in providing such meaningful accounts that the women were able to accomplish the task of respondent and complete the interview.

While Schutz and the symbolic interactionists have recognized the importance of language in the production of meanings, they have not provided any general methodological strategy for identifying the processes whereby meanings are constructed in talk (Wootton 1975). However, the ethnomethodologists, and Turner (1971), have offered such a strategy in their elucidation of the principles that guide what has become known as conversational analysis. The ethnomethodologists hold the view that it is not possible to 'extract incorrigible formulations of the meaning of talk' (Wootton 1975:94) but see the use of language as loose and imprecise. Consequently, any rendition of the meaning of talk can always be faulted since it is always possible to identify alternative interpretations. However, while talk is essentially and necessarily ambiguous, it is routinely heard by participants in a conversastion as meaningful. Ethnomethodology's main concern is with identifying the interpretive procedures involved in imputing meaning to talk. The seminal work of Garfinkel, Cicourel, and McHugh has been extended by the conversational analysts who have attempted to locate conversational structures and describe the machinery or rules whereby utterances are heard in given ways. Their basic approach is to identify speech acts within conversations and to explicate the cultural resources required to see them as such.

Here I am not so much concerned with conversation as with description and the way in which a cognitive order is accomplished. That is, with the identification of the cognitive processes and commonsense knowlege whereby events and states of affairs are categorized and recognized as part of a known order of things. This demands an ethnography of talk rather than a description of the rules presupposed in conversation.[6] While the conversational analysts provide a useful stance for approaching respondent talk the analysis here is informed more by the work of the earlier ethnomethodologists than that of these later theorists. The aim of the analysis that results from this approach is to say something about the taken-for-granted cultural resources which may be employed by individuals in their attempts to make sense of the world. It is in the description of the procedures used in constructing definitions of disorder and illness, including knowledge of persons, actions, motives, and their typical relationships, that the study attempts to make a contribution to the sociology of illness.

Notes

1. There has been some argument concerning overt versus covert approaches. The dispute centres around two issues: first, which is the more effective and, second, which is the more ethical. See Douglas (1972). These questions are only of relevance when the research setting is amenable to both kinds of approach.
2. There is research evidence which suggests that women are the main source of care for the sick within the family. See Litman (1974) for a review of relevant literature.
3. In fact there is a range of devices that may be and were employed to stimulate further talk. These include nodding, utterances such as 'uh-huh' and the like, repeating the last few words of what the respondent said, and silence.
4. See Atkinson (1978) for a discussion of this point based on Garfinkel's unpublished papers.
5. Even Blumer subscribes to this position when he says, 'Methods are mere instruments designed to identify and analyse the obdurate character of the world . . . the task of scientific activity is to lift the veils which hide or obscure what is going on' (1969:27 and 39).
6. That is, I am concerned with the analysis of interview talk about health and illness. This talk consists mainly of long descriptions of events by the respondents. Conversational analysis tends to be undertaken on short exchanges between two participants in a conversation. While interview talk may be used in this way, it is probably less fruitful than other varieties of naturally occurring talk for the location of speech acts.

3 The respondents

In this chapter I present something of what the respondents said to me about themselves and others whose health was discussed during the interviews. The aim is to provide background information about the families and the individuals concerned in order that respondents' statements reported in later chapters and my interpretation of them may be better appreciated. This information consists of basic socio-demographic data, respondents' reports of the health status of the main individuals talked about, and other matters relevant to the issues being investigated. As well as information specific to individual respondents and their respective families, I also present some of the more general themes which emerged during the interviews. The aim here is to provide a wider context within which the data may be set and to illustrate the view that the accounts given by the respondents are constructed in ways which allow them to be identified as moral persons, competent actors, and adequate performers in the social statuses to which they are assigned.[1]

Mrs P

Mrs P was interviewed six times. She was forty-four when first seen. Before her marriage she had worked in an office doing secretarial and clerical work but had given up when her children were born. Her husband was the same age and was 'a draughtsman cum office manager for an architect'. They had two children: Lindsay was eight and went to a local primary school, and Martin was four. He was due to start school within six months and was going to play-school two mornings a week.

Unlike most of the other women I interviewed Mrs P was not altogether optimistic about her family's health, 'I suppose we're sort of average really'. Referring to the children she said, 'You know these sort of childish complaints they get now and again', although at a later interview she did say, 'I suppose on the whole they are healthy. They enjoy themselves, they're out playing and everything'.

At the start of the study year Mrs P's daughter was being treated for an upper respiratory tract problem which was initially thought to be 'an allergy or hay fever'. Over the next twelve months Mrs P made frequent visits to the doctor about Lindsay's chest problem. Just prior to the third interview it had been diagnosed as bronchitis and she was prescribed antibiotics. Subsequently, she had four more courses of antibiotics when the infection returned and Mrs P began to feel that they were not getting to the root of the matter. Mrs P said, 'I got desperate in the end' and after a talk with Dr S, Lindsay was referred to an outpatient clinic. At the last interview Mrs P said Lindsay had been discharged from the clinic and told to come back if the infection returned. Mrs P thought that 'there is just that bit of a weakness with her' and said, 'I think it's unfortunate with Lindsay that she does suffer a little bit with this but on the whole she does seem to enjoy life . . . pretty active and flying around. I think possibly that I worry more about it than she does'.

Mrs P's other child, Martin, was 'pretty tough on the whole'; though he did seem to get 'a fairish number of coughs and colds through the winter' this was because he went to play-school 'and when there are so many children with colds I think when they're in a crowd they do pick them up more quickly'. At a later interview Mrs P had just received a lengthy questionnaire to complete about Martin's health before he had a medical examination at school; 'most of the things just didn't apply to him at all, he's very healthy I'm glad to say. He goes out like a light when he goes to bed and sleeps right round until seven in the morning. Then he's off again. He's so incredibly lively'.

Mrs P said that her husband's health was 'pretty good', although he was overweight. In the past he had been treated for 'a type of nervous breakdown' but 'he's got over that, he's perfectly OK now'. He had also had pneumonia twice when he was younger and Mrs P was constantly on the lookout for signs that this and the nervous breakdown were about to recur. At the second interview she said she had noticed him rubbing his chest once or twice and was going to keep an eye on him; 'I think they're things one should watch, it could be dangerous really, especially with him being overweight'. At the fourth interview Mrs P said that her husband had become depressed again and despite her attempts to persuade him he refused to go to the doctor.

Of herself, Mrs P said 'some days you feel better than others but on the whole I don't have any complaints'. She had suffered for the past ten years with a duodenal ulcer which troubled her periodically throughout the study year. She was usually able to manage the discomfort herself using a regimen that had been recommended by her brother, a fellow sufferer. Eighteen months prior to the first interview she had had an ectopic pregnancy which had been 'a bit of a shock'. She had also slipped a disc and had occasional pain from that. She said that she always felt tired 'but I'm usually on the go pretty much and I never get to bed that early'.

Mrs S

Mrs S was interviewed five times. She lived in a semi-detached house built in the 1920s, about ten minutes' walk from the doctor's surgery. At the first interview she was thirty-eight and her husband, Mike, a statistician with a large manufacturing company, was thirty-nine. They had been married for sixteen years. Their first child, Michael, was nearly six and had been physically handicapped since birth, and Joanna, their other child, was nearly three.

Like most of the others Mrs S said that herself, her husband and the children were very healthy. 'Really and truly on the whole I think I can safely say we're pretty healthy. None of us ever has a thing wrong.' Consequently, the only time they went to the doctor was for things that happened to the children. 'We can go for an awful long time without seeing him and then things crop up with the children and we go probably two or three times in a couple of months. I don't go all that much, it's mostly the children.'

According to Mrs S, Mr S couldn't be fitter, 'there's very rarely anything wrong with him', nor did he ever complain of anything. He walked to the station every morning and walked home again every evening; 'he believes in having a bit of exercise, he keeps pretty fit'. Mrs S thought that all this walking was the reason why he was so healthy. 'We haven't got a car so, you know, a lot of people seem to go down in cars, you know, as they're not as healthy as we are.' In fact, the only problem Mrs S reported for her husband in the survey year was a severe nose bleed which had happened at work. He went to the casualty department of a local hospital where the nasal membranes were cauterized and he had no further trouble.

Joanna, Mrs S's younger child, 'seems to get a lot of colds'. The main reason she ever went to the doctor was for what Mrs S called 'throat troubles'. Mrs S always took her up to Dr M 'if her throat gets bad' as she had been told that it might be necessary for her to have her tonsils out later on. The winter prior to the first interview she had had a cold almost every month, 'I've never known a girl have so many colds', and no sooner had she got rid of one she got another. Mrs S thought it was because she did not eat; 'she went through this dreadful phase of not wanting to eat. I think that was a lot to do with it. She would not sit down and eat a proper meal. I'm sure that's why she got a lot of colds'. This was a problem that. Mrs S had never had with Michael, 'he eats like a horse and that's why he's never had a cold this year'.

Michael was brain-damaged at birth, he was incontinent, could not talk or walk. Mrs S said at several interviews how healthy he was. 'Well, though he's a spastic he's healthy. I think he has a cold here and there but apart from his actual condition, you know, handicapped, I can't think of anything that he has.' A year before the first interview he had had an operation on both hips and spent six months in plaster. Of three children who had the operation at the same time, his was the only one to be a success. Mrs S had been told by the staff at the hospital that this was because he was so big and strong. Mrs S often spoke of how lucky she was:

> (Mrs S) 'I suppose I'm luckier than most that Michael isn't worse than he is. I mean I've seen so many dreadful things that I count my blessings that he's as good as he is.'

Despite the fact that he was so healthy and better off than most handicapped children he was a constant source of worry. Because of his handicap Mrs S could not take for granted his normal physical and social development. With non-handicapped children parents can assume the acquisition of skills according to a more or less predictable timetable. They can also assume the eventual independence of their offspring so that their own mortality is of limited significance. With a handicapped child these assumptions may be untenable and give rise to parental concern. On more than one occasion Mrs S said she did worry about Michael's future:

> (Mrs S) 'I worry because I think well, how's he going to be in the future. I mean, you know, is he ever going to walk, is he ever going to talk, is he ever going to be capable of . . . what happens when anything happens to my husband and I . . .'

A further source of worry for Mrs S was Michael's hip operation. She had been warned by the surgeon that it could be a failure and had seen it fail in other children:

> (Mrs S) 'It was, you know, apart from the actual operation it was the six months in plaster, you know, it was pretty nerve racking not being able to get out, worrying about Michael, was he in pain. It was in the summer and you can imagine how hot it was. So the thought that he might have to go in and have that operation again . . . we did it, we got through it yes, but to do it again would be awful.'

Consequently, Mrs S was unable to accompany Michael when he went back to hospital to have his hips checked. Her husband had to take him, 'because if they'd said that the operation had been a failure I would just have made a fool of myself, I'd probably have burst into tears or something stupid', while Mrs S stayed at home. By contrast, the six-monthly visit Michael had with his paediatrician the week before the last interview was not a source of anxiety; 'his ordinary six-monthly check-up doesn't bother me because it's just the doctor from the hospital where he was born, they watch just to keep a check on him to make sure . . . it's just a normal routine visit'. At the last interview Mrs S did say that she might worry needlessly, 'but then I'm like that, you can't change yourself can you if that's the way you are'.

Physically, Mrs S was 'very healthy', unlike most of her friends 'who always seem to be having things wrong with them'. She did say that she was always 'dead tired' but was bound to be because 'life is so hectic, there's always such a lot to do'.

Mrs G

Mrs G was interviewed three times. She was initially contacted for a pilot interview, subsequently included in the study and interviewed on two further occasions. At the time of the first contact she was seven months pregnant, and at the third and final interview had a son twelve months old. She was twenty-five and her husband was twenty-six. He worked as a contract surveyor for a large construction company.

During the last few years they had spent eighteen months in the Middle East and three months in the Caribbean while Mr G worked on company projects. Prior to her marriage Mrs G had been a teacher. She had taught while they were abroad and had only recently given up pending the birth of the child.

The Gs lived in a semi-detached house on a large estate built in the late 1960s, bought on their return from the Middle East. The estate surrounded a complex of community facilities, including the health centre where they were registered. They had joined the practice two and a half years previously when they moved into the area.

At each interview Mrs G said that she thought they were all very healthy. At one, she said, 'we've never had any serious illness at all', and at another she referred to the extent to which they needed to see the doctor:

> (Mrs G) 'Roger's never been to the doctor since we've been here, the only ailments he ever gets are common colds. I mean Daniel, obviously, he's seen the doctor on an illness basis probably three times last year. Myself, I just went for antenatal care and that's all really.'

Mrs G thought she was particularly susceptible to tonsillitis and sore throats; three out of the four visits she had made to her doctor prior to her pregnancy had been for antibiotics for her throat, although at the last interview she said, 'it's a long time . . . at least two years since I went to the doctor for that'.

Not only had Mr G never visited his doctor, Mrs G said that he never complained:

> (Int.) 'Has he never complained about his health or the way he's feeling?'

(Mrs G) 'Not really, no . . . not now, not now he's . . . he used to before he stopped smoking actually, that's the reason he did stop smoking because he felt so tired and sort of you know listless I suppose . . . since he stopped smoking he doesn't complain at all.'

Mrs G did think that this might be because his illness threshold was higher than hers:

(Mrs G) 'I would say that I was ill probably when, if Roger had the same symptom, he'd carry on, he wouldn't think he was ill.'

and this differential tendency to define symptoms as illness, a product of one's 'upbringing':

(Mrs G) 'Probably if you've had parents that made a fuss over an illness, sort of treated it as a severe thing each time, er . . . you'd feel different than if you had parents that sort of said you're alright, get your coat on and off to school.'

Despite the fact that they were all healthy, Mrs G did not think that they were any better or worse than any of the other families that they knew, 'we're just similar really'. Apart from making sure that they had a varied diet she took no other precautions to maintain their health, 'we just accept things and deal with them as they come'.

Mrs F

Mrs F was interviewed four times. At the first contact she was forty-six and a housewife. Prior to giving up work she had been a school secretary for eight years and spent two years as an educational welfare officer. Mr F was also forty-six and a liaison engineer for an industrial concern making car instruments. The Fs had two daughters: Clare was fifteen and still at school, Madge was seventeen and had done two jobs since leaving school.

When I asked Mrs F about her family's health she said her husband was 'very healthy' and her daughters 'very fit'. She went on, 'That's what worries me about joining in your survey, really I don't feel we're the right family'. Mr F rarely saw the doctor and 'never has time off work unless he's dying'. Her elder daughter, 'she's on the pill, that's the only thing she goes for, to twist his arm and say she must have it'. The younger daughter 'has had one or two bouts of sort of, she gets these swollen glands and sort of a slight temperature. I have had the doctor round a couple of times when she's had a high temperature and I've kept her in bed, but as I say, it's very seldom'.

Mrs F herself was 'pretty fit'. 'The only reason I've been to the doctor which was three months ago I had a sort of eczema of the outer ear, but that has cleared up.' Mrs F did, however, suffer from allergic attacks in which her face and her eyes in particular became swollen and painful. Despite numerous tests it had never been definitely diagnosed as an allergy nor had an agent which was responsible been identified. Mrs F had been told to live with it and usually managed occurrences herself. It bothered her periodically throughout the study.year.

Although Mrs F thought that her family were healthy she did not think this made them unusual in any way:

> (Mrs F) 'I just thought we were too healthy to be involved in the sort of, er, census that you're doing. I felt you would have liked a family who succumbed to all sorts of things . . . who had all sorts of peculiar er . . . regular ailments. No, I don't necessarily think we're that healthy, there are plenty of healthy people about. I just felt we were too healthy for you to be bothered with.'

One problem Mrs F talked about at all four interviews was her mother. At one interview she said, 'I think there's more to tell you about my mother than there is about the rest of us'. Mrs F's mother was eighty-four and living on her own 'trying to cope and not be a burden to anyone'. Mrs F saw her several times a week to take her shopping, to collect her pension, or to see relatives. 'She's more or less housebound except when I take her out.'

Mr and Mrs F and both daughters were heavily involved with and committed to a number of local amateur dramatic companies. At one interview Mrs F said, 'we do amateur theatricals, we're up to our necks in amateur theatricals'. Much of their spare time was taken up with this activity and Mrs F often said how busy they all were: 'You know, we lead such busy lives we haven't got time to be ill or to go to the doctor's unless it's really desperate'. Much of what Mrs F said about her own and her family's health was related to this interest. For example, when talking about the precautions they took regarding their health Mrs F went on:

> (Mrs F) 'As I say, if it's vital for us to be well we do take extra precautions, it's only for shows that we care about being ill.'

Mrs N

Mrs N was interviewed three times. She was forty-three at the first interview and a housewife. Her husband was forty-five and a manager with an investment company dealing in property bonds. They had two daughters: Tina was seventeen and Lesley was fourteen.

At the first interview Mrs N said that her family's health was excellent: 'they only just have minor things, a headache or . . . unless something crops up they're not really unhealthy at all'. She went on, 'I'm more nervous than the rest of them, I mean I see Dr . . . I see him mostly because of that'. Mrs N described herself as a 'natural worrier' and found her family's health a cause for concern:

> (Mrs N) 'I must say I'm the type of person that anything more than a headache does give me a hell of a lot of worry, you know, I'm happy when everything goes smoothly but obviously something crops up and then I do worry terribly.'

Later in the interview she said 'Thank goodness we're a pretty healthy family so there's not really any problems . . . my mother's the only source of worry because of the operations and troubles she has'.

Mr N suffered from recurrent headaches. At each of the interviews he was said by Mrs N to be complaining. Mrs N thought it was due to hard work and said there was 'a lot of strain' attached to his job. He had been prescribed Valium and sleeping pills by the doctor but these had not stopped him getting them. The elder daughter had had nothing more serious than her tonsils out and was currently in pain because her wisdom teeth were erupting. Mrs N's younger daughter had only recently returned to school after having glandular fever, 'she had it very mildly which was very lucky'. Mrs N described her as obstinate and said she was going through 'an awkward phase'.

Mrs R

Mrs R was interviewed five times. She was interviewed alone except for the second occasion when her husband was present. At the time of the first contact Mrs R was thirty-three. She was a housewife, although one morning a week she worked outside the home doing bookkeeping and secretarial work. Mr R was thirty-six and a director of a charity. The Rs had two children: Lee was six and Alison eight.

At the first interview Mrs R said that her own health was excellent: 'Generally, I feel very well. I've had one or two things, obviously, but on the whole I usually feel very well'. Almost a year before this first interview Mrs R had an operation to remove the root of a tooth from her sinus where it had been causing an infection. The operation had not been entirely successful since Mrs R still had occasional facial pain. 'I haven't had it lately so maybe it's clearing up. I'm a great optimist, I keep hoping things will clear up.'

Mrs R said that her daughter's health was 'pretty good', although she had recently gone through a period when she had complained frequently of abdominal pain. The problem had never been diagnosed because the doctor had been unwilling to subject the child to investigation. Mrs R had thought 'she might be becoming a bit of a hypochondriac'. Mrs R's son 'has had problems almost all his life. He suffered from tonsilitis from the age of three months very severely. It fizzled out when he was four, just before we changed to Dr M. He still gets a lot of coughs, colds and earache . . . which is a bit of a problem with him because I do worry about his ears'. When Mrs R was asked at one interview if either of the children had been to the doctor in the previous four weeks she said, 'I should think my son has about his ears, this would apply at almost any time. He does have to go fairly frequently'. Other than that, Mrs R said that he was 'all right'.

A few weeks before the first interview Mr R had visited his doctor complaining of depression and had been prescribed antidepressants. At several interviews throughout the study year Mrs R spoke of her husband as being her biggest problem: 'my husband is the only real problem . . . what the rest of us have had is nothing'. Though his condition deteriorated during the year, at the last interview Mrs R was hopeful about his future.

Mr R had originally been treated for depression in 1968, 'that was just sort of limited treatment on Valium, that's all I did have at that time'. Although the antidepressants he had been prescribed by the doctor seemed to have a beneficial effect initially 'in the end they were not successful'. By the time of the second interview Mr R had been referred to a psychiatrist and later Mrs R complained about the doctor's reluctance to make the referral which they had finally had to demand. Because the first experience with psychotropics had been 'pretty disastrous' Mr R refused further drugs and was put on the waiting list for group therapy.

During the middle part of the study year, while waiting to join a therapy group, Mr R had become considerably worse. He was finally admitted to a group after Mrs R phoned the hospital to say that he was no longer able to face work. Initially, the group therapy seemed to be useful and Mr R went back to work although after attending three or four sessions he stopped going to work altogether. Mr and Mrs R then went back to Dr M and asked to see the psychiatrist again, and after a wait of four weeks they received an appointment. The psychiatrist recommended in-patient treatment and Mr R was admitted for two and a half weeks. He spent a further week as an out-patient and then returned to work.

After the hospital treatment there had been a 'steady improvement' though Mrs R did add 'he's better than he was, he's got a long way to go, he's not cured as yet'. She was, in fact, surprised by the progress he had made, 'it's faster than I thought it would be, I thought it would take a lot longer than it seems to be doing', but was unsure as to how complete a recovery he would make.

Despite her husband's continuing problem and her anticipation that it would only be solved in the long term, Mrs R was not too pessimistic about her family:

(Mrs R) 'I think on the whole we are healthy apart from my husband's problem. I would say that we are quite a healthy family, erm . . . my husband's physically healthy, I wouldn't say we were an ailing family at all, erm . . . we don't have anything that causes any real worry other than my husband's problem. No, I think we're fine.'

Some aspects of the everyday life of wives and mothers

The above descriptions are sketches of the contexts upon which disorders of various kinds intrude and within which they are managed. While each of these contexts is specific, in the sense that each family is a unique social unit and each individual within it unique in terms of biography and life experiences, certain features of those contexts are shared. Though individuals, the respondents were all women, wives, and mothers. That is, they all occupied a number of related social statuses by means of which their experiences may be typified.[2] What is known about those statuses provides the respondents with a vocabulary for describing their experiences in ways which renders them common.

As Chapters 4, 5, and 6 will reveal, these statuses may be important for two reasons. Firstly, they or what is associated with them may be invoked to account for various problematic experiences and the actions taken to deal with them. Irrespective of whether occupancy of these statuses does act as a constraint on action by limiting choice or other means, they may be presented as so doing in explanations of what was or was not done. Secondly, some of what was said by the respondents in the interviews may be read as demonstrations of adequate performance in these statuses. Voysey (1975) has argued that there exists an 'official morality of family life' by means of which parental performance may be judged. For example, adequate performance in the role of wife and mother requires success as the manager of family and household and the fulfilment of the material and psychological needs of children. The women themselves used these and related criteria in criticizing the performance of others. They also reported feeling guilty when their own performance did not meet the requirements they set:

(Mrs R) '[When my husband gets depressed] I get impatient all round and instead of being more patient with the children I'm less and then I get guilty about what I'm doing to them.'

In this way, the respondents' descriptions of their own families and their own conduct in particular are expressions of this official morality.

More fundamentally, however, the women I interviewed are 'persons' (Puccetti 1968) and 'members' (Garfinkel 1967). Puccetti has argued that the ascription of personhood requires that an object is accorded both an intellectual and a moral character. According to Voysey, this presupposes 'access to and familiarity with a conceptual scheme' and 'the ability to assimilate a conceptual scheme in which moral words and phrases have a place' (1975:31). Garfinkel's notion of member involves the possession of natural language and a body of culturally accredited knowledge. Where a moral character is not imputed, the individual concerned may not be viewed as a person. Children are temporary non-persons since their moral characters are assumed to be in the process of formation. Similarly, the mentally handicapped and the mentally ill may be viewed in these terms; since it is assumed that they are not capable of making moral decisions because of an inherent or acquired defect, they are not usually held responsible for their actions. Children and the mentally handicapped may also be viewed as non-members, as incompetents, given their limited access to and use of natural language and the stock of knowledge necessary for making adequate sense of the world. The behaviour of children, the mentally ill, and the mentally handicapped may be interpreted as the inevitable product of the categories they occupy. As Voysey says, parents 'know what children in general are like' and may use this knowledge to make sense of their own children's behaviour. Similarly, behaviour which appears 'senseless' may be comprehended when it is learned that the agents of that behaviour were children. For example, in talking to Mrs P prior to my final interview with her, I was describing how the offices where I worked had been broken into and property stolen. The following week there was a second break-in when some of the property stolen at the first was returned:

(Mrs P) 'The same lot came back?'
(Int.) 'Yes, but it was only children.'
(Mrs P) 'Oh, well.'

Subsequently, Mrs P went on to describe a series of break-ins at the local church hall:

(Mrs P) 'They left it in an absolute shambles. And when they got in last week they threw black paint all over the floor and all down the walls as well. It's upsetting really because I mean, gosh, for a church you don't expect this really. I don't know, but it does seem ridiculous doesn't it? There again, I'm sure it's children.'

In both of these cases apparently irrational actions are understandable as the actions of children. Children's behaviour is not, then, to be interpreted in terms of the motives assumed to inform adult conduct. As non-persons and non-competents they cannot be judged in terms of the criteria by which persons and competents may be judged since they are not assumed to be rational actors. Similar actions on the part of adults may be seen as the symptoms of mental illness since they cannot be explained in terms of culturally acceptable motives (Morgan 1975).

That children are considered to be non-persons and non-competents has implications for the parental role. Firstly, parents may be held to constitute the moral character of their children in so far as they are held responsible for his or her behaviour. The behaviour of a child reflects on that of the parents such that deviant or aberrant conduct on the part of a child may be interpreted as an indicator of moral defect in the parents. Mrs P, talking about local children who used bad language and were generally rowdy and ill-mannered, said:

> (Mrs P) 'One time they called out abuse to me and I turned round and said just watch what you're up to, but, erm, you can't do much about it, I don't suppose if their parents don't bother, you don't stand much chance.'

Even where a child's 'deviance' is non-motivated, as in the case of a handicapped child, the parents may be held responsible or may feel that their moral character is threatened. Davis and Strong, in a study of clinics for assessing the development of potentially handicapped children, suggest that:

> 'one possible effect of such testing is to call into question the motivation and competence of the parents. When a child is compared with an "ideal type" there is always the possibility that discrepancies between the particular child's development and the ideal type can be explained in terms of the quality of the family. Therefore, there is considerable pressure on the parents to have their child accepted as normal and thereby get their own normality confirmed.' (Davis and Strong 1976:157)

Secondly, parents are held responsible for providing an environment that satisfies the material, social, and emotional needs of their children. Inadequate parenthood consists in failing to provide for these needs. Given that any competent adult is assumed to be capable of adequate parenthood on the basis of knowledge acquired through socialization and personal experience of family life, such failure is a further indicator of moral defect. Alternatively, it may call for an account by means of which failure may be justified.

The significance attached to a 'normal family life' is evidenced by the fact that a family life identified as deficient in some way is often accorded a causal role in the genesis of delinquency, mental illness, and deviance of other kinds. One needs only to refer to the maternal deprivation thesis, the association of delinquency and broken homes, and Laing's work on the origins of schizophrenia. Underlying these there is some notion of 'needs' which must be satisfied if normal social and psychological development is to take place. The failure to satisfy children's needs may then be invoked to account for aberrant behaviour on their part and employed to construct a criticism of parents' actions. When Mrs S's daughter was badly bitten by a boy at nursery school, Mrs S was able to find an explanation in the character of his family life:

> (Mrs S) 'I don't know if it's anything to do with it but his mother, both her and her husband play for a symphony orchestra and of course they're never at home, they've had a succession of au pair girls and now they've got a permanent nanny so you just wonder if it might be something to do with that, you know, you know what children are like, they get a bit funny if they haven't got mother there all the time. I don't care what anybody says there's no substitute for a mum.'

Here Mrs S explains the boy's behaviour as a product of an absentee mother. As she said later, 'I don't know whether it's just something that Simon's lacking at home, you know, because they're going away to Japan for three weeks in May to play with the orchestra'. Contained in the account are assumptions about what children are like, in terms of the way they may respond to situations, and also about their need for a mother. Not just any female will do; au pairs and nannies 'are no substitute for a mum'. This, of course, carries implications for a mother's role in that it identifies appropriate conduct for one who occupies that category.

It is not only a child's behaviour that may bring about moral condemnation of parents, other observable indicators may be taken as evidence of parental neglect. Later in the interview Mrs S expressed concern about the interpretations to which the bruising resulting from the boy's biting may be subject:

> (Mrs S) 'I'm worried about the marks it's left, they're taking an awful long time to heal. I can imagine when she starts school they'll think I've been ill-treating her. I'm quite worried about that.'

As Davis and Strong point out, our notion of the nature of children requires that they be treated in a special way by adults, such that their maltreatment is seen as particularly reprehensible. This is reflected in the legal system whereby crimes against children are more heavily penalized than crimes against adults. Similarly, ill-treatment of a child by a parent is an especially condemnable form of inadequate parenthood. Hence, Mrs S's concern lest a formal authority suspect that she be guilty of this misdemeanour.

One of the functions of the family is the care of children and part of that care involves the maintenance of health. An absence of health in a child may cast doubt on the adequacy of parental care. This is particularly so if those routine procedures assumed to contribute to good health are not implemented. When Mrs G was talking about a neighbour's child who was always ill she commented: 'Well, I often see him without a hat on or anything like that so, you know . . .'.

Underlying statements of this kind are theories about what contributes
to good health. These theories provide the basis for action on the part of a
mother in caring for her child. Typically, the practices derived from these
theories involved making sure the child had a good and varied diet and
keeping it warm if it was cold. The women I interviewed were identifiable
as good mothers since they knew of these theories and acted accordingly:

(Mrs S) 'I like to make sure that they eat well, I think that's very
important that they go out with a good breakfast in the morning. I
think, erm, you know, if they went out on an empty stomach they
might not be so fit.'

(Mrs P) 'If they've not been well I do give them a bit of a tonic, some
vitamin drops and a bit of extra stuff like that or make sure they eat a bit
of extra fruit and things you know. They have vitamin drops every
morning through the autumn and winter months right through to late
spring. Most of my friends seem to give their children something you
know.'

(Mrs G) 'I keep him well wrapped up if it's cold, you know, a warm
jumper on and a warm coat, that sort of thing.'

These precautions are not to be seen as the actions of overprotective or
fussy mothers; rather, they constitute the routine activities of a mother in
caring for a child. Mrs S indicated as much when she stated that she did
not believe in 'mollycoddling':

(Mrs S) 'We don't mollycoddle, I don't believe in mollycoddling
children but, erm, just the normal care that you would take, you know,
the way our parents did.'

While it is important that mothers take normal care, it is also important
that such care is not exaggerated. Mrs P, in attempting to solve the
dilemma of her daughter suffering recurrent respiratory infections
despite her routine care, identified the possible consequences of being
over-protective:

(Mrs P) 'I sometimes think perhaps well really the more you try and
coddle them up perhaps the worse off they are. Often the more you try
and take care of them they seem worse off, I don't know.'

However, Mrs P did say that she tried not to fuss over them, 'I let them
go out and get plenty of fresh air and enjoy themselves'. Consequently,
her failure may lie in the invalidity of the theories she employed in her
attempts to keep her children healthy:

(Mrs P) 'It's amazing some of these children that play out. I've seen them in all weathers, they seem to be out with no big coats on, they seem to be as tough as old boots.'

Despite evidence such as this which suggests that the theories of health maintenance employed by mothers are incorrect, it is likely that the actions to which they give rise will be continued. Such actions have a symbolic as well as a practical value. As indicators of parental concern, they allow others to identify mothers as providing proper care. That there is a consensus about these matters was suggested by Mrs P when she said, 'Most of my friends seem to give their children something'.

While parents are held to be responsible for their children's health, it is inevitable that children do fall ill. For this not to reflect on the character of them as parents some of the women I interviewed pointed out that there were limits to parental control. As Mrs R explained, children are to a certain extent independent and, for some of the time, outside parental supervision:

(Mrs R) 'Although you try to keep them clean and everything at home all right, you never know when they're not in the house or where they go or exactly what they do.'

At another interview, Mrs P invoked the nature of children as a constraint on her ability to provide the sort of care she thought appropriate:

(Mrs P) 'You air their clothes and try and see they're warmly dressed up and they come flying out of school with coats half buttoned up and perhaps it's raining, you know, but well, that's kids, you can't stop them.'

Eventually, children reach an age when they will not allow parents to exercise control. Moreover, once they are at a stage of life where they are accorded the status of persons and competents, parents may reasonably abdicate their responsibility, so that failures of health reflect on the individual concerned and not the parent. Mrs F, talking about her seventeen-year-old daughter said:

(Mrs F) 'She won't go to the dentist, she's an individual you know, can't be bothered, you're not allowed to look after her, she's a big girl now. Anyway, last week she was having pain so she did have to go. It was more or less an emergency, but it was her own fault for leaving it so long.'

In these cases parental responsibility may be fulfilled by providing adequate warning of the consequences of certain actions. At the second interview Mrs N talked about her younger daughter who was having to have a lot of fillings. She went on, 'In her younger days too many sweets and sickly things, but then you see she's rather obstinate, when she wants to eat it she would go ahead and do it. I was always warning her about it'.

As I have mentioned above, parents are held to be responsible for their conduct as parents on the basis of the assumption that any adult is capable of an adequate performance in that role. That is, it is assumed that an adult will know of what is involved in bringing up a child and be motivated to act accordingly. It is expected that ordinary experience provides the opportunity for individuals to acquire knowledge about children, their needs, and how to fulfil them. It is also expected that parents will acquire knowledge of their own children as a result of interaction with them so that what Voysey calls 'normal recipes of child rearing' may be adapted where necessary to the individual child. State-ments illustrating both of these points were made by Mrs S during my interviews with her. The first is taken from an exchange where Mrs S was telling me how she preferred to deal with her children's problems herself rather than bothering the doctor:

> (Mrs S) 'I would never call the doctor out unless it was really serious, you know, for us but if it was the children and I thought they really should come then I would do. I wouldn't, you know, just leave them to it sort of thing. But if it's something I can sort out myself then I'll do that. I mean I think it comes naturally to a parent to a mum to know what to do for your child if they're poorly.'

The second is taken from an exchange where Mrs S was describing how Michael, her handicapped son, was sometimes brought home from nursery school looking pale and unwell. Mrs S thought it might be due to his being strapped incorrectly and uncomfortably in his wheelchair:

> (Mrs S) 'When he's with me he's never ill 'cos I know what I'm doing with him.'

For Mrs S her competence in managing her children's problems is a product of her status as a parent, a natural consequence of motherhood. It is also enhanced by her specific knowledge of her own children such that she is able to provide for their particular needs. Consequently, when Michael went into hospital for his operation, Mrs S stayed with him:

> (Mrs S) 'He went in for nine days to have the operation. I stayed in with him which I'm glad I did, he needed me, you know. Some people said, Oh you're silly, you've got Joanna, but I think he needed me more than she did, she had Mike at home looking after her and he, well, he had nobody and he's a helpless child and he can't communicate. I know everything that he needs and what he wants so it helped the nurses too.'

The special knowledge that mothers employ in dealing with their children's problems may also be used in dealing with the problems of other family members. Wives, for example, may acquire an intimate knowledge of their husbands which allows them to recognize when all is not well. Mrs R said that she always knew when her husband was going through one of his depressed phases although others may not have been able to recognize this:

> (Mrs R) 'Usually he becomes very quiet, doesn't want to talk, he can't bear any kind of noise . . . I can tell just by his face, just by looking at him. Maybe that's because I know him so well, I don't know if anybody else could, to me his face seems to change, he just looks thoroughly miserable.'

Having recognized such a phase, Mrs R was able to take action to 'slow the pace of life down' and shield him from routine family business. Although the knowledge acquired through her status as wife and intimate allowed Mrs R to identify when her husband was not well, limits to her competence to help were imposed by this and other statuses. At the last interview Mrs R talked at length about the group therapy her husband was receiving for his depression. He thought that it might be contributing to his depression and Mrs R was unsure that it was having a beneficial effect. However, she was quite keen for him to continue attending the sessions:

> (Mrs R) 'If it doesn't itself do any good it's a place he can go and talk things out other than with me. Obviously, I'm too involved to be very much good to him and besides I haven't got the knowledge.'

Here, Mrs R invoked her status as a wife to explain her inability to be of help to her husband. As an intimate she is 'too involved' to be of much use, unlike the disinterested professionals and fellow sufferers Mr R met at his group therapy sessions. Though the group which Mr R was currently attending did not seem to be leading to an improvement in his psychiatric state, the group therapy sessions he experienced as an in-patient had enabled him to 'recognize a lot about himself'. As an interested party Mrs R was not able to be objective about his situation or the origins of his depression and was unlikely to contribute to this process of learning about himself. In addition, Mrs R claims to be limited by her status as a lay individual, as someone who does not have the knowledge or experience to provide a solution to this particular problem.

Thus, while mothers did assert that they were competent to deal with the health problems of their respective families, they did recognize that there were limits to that competence. These limits were sometimes offered as justifications for seeking expert help. Mrs G, for example, said on more than one occasion that she would only consult the doctor about problems that she could not handle herself. As Schutz indicates, an individual's recipe for achieving his practical purpose at hand tells him when it is necessary to consult an expert. The inadequacy of commonsense knowledge is both recognized and accepted by the lay actor given the existence of professional problem solvers. Consequently, mothers are not expected nor do they expect to be able to handle all the problems that may arise, since some require the attention of those who possess specialist knowledge. However, they may be expected to be able to recognize when a child is unwell and when it is necessary to seek the advice of an expert. As Mrs R said: 'I'm reasonably confident I would recognize if there were anything wrong, I'd only get worried if there were anything unusual or something unexpected happened to one.'

However, as I will argue in Chapter 6, the problem is not necessarily this simple. The ambiguity surrounding problematic experiences frequently presented the women I interviewed with a problem, that of deciding whether they were dealing with a routine or trivial disorder, or with something needing expert attention. Where children were concerned, they often chose to be 'on the safe side' and consulted the doctor for his opinion.

As mothers, the women I interviewed expected their children to be a routine and continuing source of trouble and anxiety. In fact, worrying about the children was presented as a natural and inevitable consequence of being a parent: 'I do worry about the children. I think everybody does. It wouldn't be natural if you didn't worry about the children' (Mrs S).

Later in the interview Mrs S emphasized the same point: 'Of course you worry about them. I think you would do unless there's something inhuman about you and you just didn't care.'

For Mrs S anxiety about her children's welfare is an ever-present fact of life common to all parents such that it is only the pathological who could fail to be worried. For Mrs N, worrying about her children was also a fact of life until they got to the stage where they had outgrown the problems normally associated with childhood:

(Mrs N) 'You find you have more problems when they're toddlers. I had my hair falling out . . . but I'm older and wiser, much better because I think they're past chicken pox, they've both had their glandular fever, they're past this, they're past that, you know.'

That things would be better when her children were older was not anticipated by Mrs S, however:

(Mrs S) 'From what I've been told, you worry more. Everybody that has got older children says as they get older you worry about them, erm, there just seems to be more problems one after the other, they say they're better when they're young like this.'

Mr S's brother had a daughter of fifteen and a son of eighteen and he 'worries just as much about them now', and her next-door neighbour 'she's got a married daughter and a son in South Africa and she still worries about them'. Accounts by others of their experiences of parenthood thus allow Mrs S to construct a conception of her own future *vis-à-vis* the problems that she can anticipate.[3] For her, the normal problems of childhood give way to the normal problems of adolescence and so on, 'You worry about them as long as you've got them'.

The accounts of others not only allow mothers to anticipate that child rearing will be fraught with problems, they also enable them to interpret the problems they do encounter as typical experiences of motherhood:

(Mrs S) 'Sometimes I find that everything gets on top of me, the children get too much, Joanne she can be a little so and so, you know, like they all can at three years old and I've warned the next door neighbour, she's been exactly the same she said, she, you know, used to feel the same with her children when she was young, so I said, don't take any notice of me if you hear me having a good scream, it's just getting it out of my system and I feel much better then.'

The typicality of experiences of this kind is also reinforced if they can be seen to stem from the nature of children:

(Mrs S) 'You can't take it out on your children . . . children are children, they get naughty, they get bored, I do know some people take it out on their children but I wouldn't want to do that.'

Thus, a conception of what children are like and assumptions about the typicality of her response means that Mrs S can constitute these experiences as 'normal family life' rather than as indicators of family pathology.

As I mentioned earlier, a pathological family life is assumed to be the cause of various types of pathology in its members. Children in particular are viewed as being vulnerable to abnormalities in family life such that when family troubles do occur attempts are often made to conceal this from them by the presentation of a normal front. At two interviews Mrs R made statements about the possibility of her husband's depression having an adverse effect on the children:

(Mrs R) 'I get worried about the children, whether it's going to have an effect on them, as they see he's not quite as he should be.'

(Mrs R) 'I've been very worried about them. Well, you know, we told them that he's tired and that he needs to rest which I don't really like doing because I don't want them to get the idea that their father's an invalid, I don't think that's very good for them. I haven't wanted to tell them exactly what's wrong because I think that could worry them very much.'

In these statements Mrs R claims that the identification of their father as deficient in some way will be harmful to her children. That is, their assumed need for a normal father will not be met and this will have untoward consequences. Mrs R is anxious to avoid telling them exactly what is wrong with their father since 'that could worry them'; at the same time she is worried about the explanation she offers for her husband's symptoms since it may lead them to identify him as 'an invalid' which, given the need for a normal father, is not very good for them. Mrs P also expressed concern about her husband's depression and tried to conceal this from the children by normalizing his symptoms:

(Mrs P) 'I get worried about the children, they keep saying to me, "What's the matter with daddy?", and I say, "Well he's rather upset, he's over-tired and he's not too well", you know, and you sort of pass it off, but it does get a bit difficult at times.'

Mrs R also supplied her children with a normalizing explanation of her husband's problem and went on to express doubts about whether they had fully accepted it:

(Mrs R) 'When he went into hospital we told them that he'd overworked, he has in fact worked very hard over the past years, and that all the work had made him very tired and he needed a long rest and he was going into hospital. And I think they. accepted it er . . . I think, one can never be very sure because I think children notice more than one gives them credit for and they don't always speak about it, they pretend to accept things sometimes without . . . perhaps I think they're afraid to stir things up.'

Mrs R's doubts about the success of her attempts at concealment stem from her conception of the nature of children. That is, children are often wise to situations to a greater extent that their ascribed status as incompetents would allow. Their sensitivity to trouble in the family may be hidden from others by their pretence to accept adult versions of the world and reluctance to challenge that version by speaking about it. Their response to Mrs R's explanation cannot then be taken as an indicator of their failure to see through her account since they are equally capable of the presentation of a normal front. Consequently, 'one can never be sure'.

General conceptions of what children are like thus render problematic the management of troubles such as parental illness and may create the kinds of dilemma Mrs R describes. Such conceptions also inform parental responses to the more mundane problems of child rearing that may be encountered. Mrs S, in managing her young daughter's refusal to eat, made recourse to commonsense knowledge about children:

(Mrs S) 'I didn't force her or make a fuss because I don't think that's right.'I think the more you make a fuss the more they get awkward, you know, they play you up which is very true they do. I just didn't take any notice. I'd put it on the table and if she didn't eat it I'd take it away again . . . but I thought we'd get it over and done with eventually.'

The possession of a stock of such recipes for coping with various aspects of family life enables mothers to respond in ways which may be considered to be appropriate. In the context of interaction with others accounts which draw on these accepted recipes enable them to construct and maintain a good identity. As I have argued in Chapter 2, a research interview, where mothers are questioned directly about their management of family problems, is one context where such an identity may be reaffirmed. I assume then that the accounts that the women I interviewed gave were constructed in ways which allow them to be seen to conform to socially accepted criteria defining good performance in given social roles. I also assume that their descriptions of their own conduct or other aspects of the world around them are displays of their personhood and their membership. That is, these descriptions provide for the interpretation of their actions as the conduct of moral actors behaving in ways that might reasonably be expected of anyone in given circumstances. They also demonstrate their access to a culturally accredited stock of knowledge which they are able to employ to make reasonable sense of their experience of the world. In making reasonable sense they are able to present those experiences as part of a normal order of things.

In this chapter I have presented some descriptive data about the respondents and their families. I have also presented data to illustrate some aspects of what might be called the everyday life of wives and mothers. In particular, I have attempted to describe something of their conceptions of children, their own role as wives and mothers, and their notions of the normal experience of motherhood and family life. In the following chapters I will be concerned with three issues: the way in which the women made sense of problematic experiences by locating them within a medical frame of reference, the construction of definitions of illness, and accounts of the way in which signs and symptoms are practically managed. These three themes constitute important aspects of what I have termed a management sequence.

Notes

1. In the data fragments reproduced in this and the following chapters, 'Int.' means interviewer and refers to the author. Data in this chapter are for background information only; in Chapters 4 to 6 however data fragments are referred to on more than one occasion and have been numbered for ease of cross-reference.

2. Mrs S, talking about one of her close friends, described some of the common features of their life situation:

> (Mrs S) 'I see her sort of every day, you know. She's the same age as me, she's got three youngsters, you know, we've a lot in common and I think she and I talk more than anybody really about our health problems. We're very much alike in a lot of ways, we suffer from the same sorts of things, you know, nerves, the children . . . We met each other when we went to relaxation classes for our first children and, erm, we always talk things over as regards ourselves, our children and, you know, it helps.'

3. The experiences of others are often used in constructing definitions of events and making projections about what will happen in the future. For example, Mrs R was uncertain about how well her husband was progressing following discharge from in-patient psychiatric treatment because his condition seemed to fluctuate from day to day. Mrs R was able to make sense of this by drawing on the experience of a friend:

> (Mrs R) 'It's a very long struggle . . . because I think I told you about a friend of ours who had a bad breakdown and I saw the wife the other day when I'd had rather a trying day and I said it really is tough and she said you don't have to tell me. After her husband was discharged from hospital it took eighteen months she said, to get back to any kind of normality, she said eighteen months of sheer hell. So obviously, it's just a long-term thing and you can't put a time to it.'

Consequently, Mrs R was able to construe what was happening to her husband as typical for this kind of problem.

4 Making sense of problematic experience

In managing problematic experiences of any kind there are several problems facing an actor that must be solved with the cognitive and material resources at his disposal. He must be able to recognize departures from some state considered usual or routine for himself or others. He must employ some stock of knowledge to assess the significance of those departures and to formulate plans of action to deal with them. He must be able to realize those plans, evaluate their outcome, and, if necessary, formulate alternatives, and he must be able to employ interactional skills in order to deal with the individuals he encounters in his attempt to solve his problems. Because others may challenge the way these cognitive and practical problems are managed, he must also be able to construct rationales to justify what he thought and what he did.

Problematic experiences are subject to interpretive work so that they may be defined and classified. The practical management of these experiences may depend upon the outcome of this interpretive activity. In some instances, however, an individual may not be able to make sense of an experience in the light of the knowledge available to him. In these cases action may be as much directed towards identifying the nature of the experience as seeking its resolution. Where an individual's knowledge is inadequate to make experience consistent with a familiar world then he may resort to consulting others, including professional problem solvers, who may offer solutions to the cognitive and practical problems with which he is faced.

The importance of finding a solution to the cognitive problems posed by problematic experience has been graphically described by Cunningham (1978) and Burton (1975). Cunningham has documented the difficulties faced by multiple sclerosis sufferers prior to being offered a diagnosis which would allow them to make sense of their symptoms and organize an appropriate response. Similarly, Burton's study of families with a chronically sick child reveals the anxieties suffered by mothers who had noticed a discrepancy between their baby's progress and what they assumed to be normal development. It was often many months before they acquired a diagnostic label for the child's condition despite consultations with their doctor and demands for paediatric referral. It can also be illustrated by some of the data I collected.

Mrs S was the mother of a disabled child. She had told me at the first interview of some of the problems she faced: 'If I ever go to the doctor's it's my nerves, having Michael, you know'. At the third interview she elaborated on this while describing a problem she had been having with her breathing:

(S1) (Mrs S) 'Well, I had to go to the doctor's 'cos I . . . Oh, yes, that's what you want to know about probably, more than anything . . . nerves, this is me. I went oh for about two weeks, I think about two, it was before Christmas I couldn't get my breath properly, you know, I was gasping for breath, it was a most horrible feeling. I've still got it and, erm, at least I know what it is now, it's not so bad, and, erm, I thought at first it didn't bother me too much and it gradually got worse so I thought I'd better go and see the doctor. I'd no idea what it was. Anyway, he took my blood pressure, that was all right, my heart was fine, so he said what he thought it was just nerves, you know, just a bad attack of bad nerves as he phrased it. So he just gave me some tablets and I took those which really didn't make any difference but at least I felt better because I knew what it was. You know, I mean I think you worry far more if you think it might be your heart or something like that, than if you do nerves, at least I do. I mean you might say well why have I got nerves, but I think it's because of having a handicapped child, you know.'

Here, the doctor's diagnosis not only provided a label for Mrs S's experience, it also allowed her to make sense of it in terms of her biography as the mother of a handicapped child. For Mrs S, suffering with her nerves was part of the usual order of things. She had had a variety of problems in the past and expected that these would continue and that she would be able to cope with them when they arose. Defining the breathing problem as a manifestation of her nerves not only ruled out a series of alternatives, 'your heart or something like that', it routinized it as something a person in her life situation might reasonably expect. The diagnosis of bad nerves told her what was wrong and in this instance told her why she had it, since a link had already been constructed between her nerves and relevant features of her biography. In this way something unknown, potentially dangerous, and worrying became assimilated into a familiar order. As Mrs S put it later in the interview, 'it was funny you know as soon as I talked to him [the doctor] about it and he told me what it was I felt better'. Despite the fact that the tablets prescribed by the doctor had very little effect Mrs S did not return to the doctor with the problem during the period in which I continued to interview her.

These data also demonstrate that answers to at least two questions have to be found to achieve a sense of order. The first, 'What is wrong?', is often answered by a lay or medical diagnosis. The second, 'Why has this happened?', requires the construction of an explanation to account for the event or experience in question. It is sometimes the case that one or both of these questions remains unanswered. While scientific medicine or commonsense knowledge may provide diagnoses to confirm the suspicion that something is wrong, an explanation of what has happened may not be forthcoming (Burton 1975). Alternatively, diagnoses may not be available, so that the nature and meaning of an event is never determined.

In the remainder of this chapter I will expand on these issues by an examination of the way the women I interviewed went about classifying and explaining some of the problematic experiences with which they were confronted. The data consists of the women's accounts of how they decided that something was wrong with themselves or a member of their family and how they were able to make sense of this by locating the cause and determining the significance of the disorder in question.

Recognizing disorder: types of cue

Problematic experiences can be defined as events, situations, or states of affairs which disturb the taken-for-granted attitude towards the world and call for interpretive and explanatory activity. These experiences may follow from changes in the biological state of the body, either 'pathological' changes such as those caused by disease, or changes associated with normal physiological mechanisms. These changes must manifest themselves in some way available to experience. Physiological states such as hypertension may not be discovered because they do not intrude on the everyday experience of the body. Alternatively, problematic experiences may arise from changes in the social functioning of an individual. Judgements of mental illness, for example, hinge entirely on behavioural 'abnormalities' such as disordered behaviour, perception, or thought. These states of affairs may be viewed as problematic by the individual concerned or the others with whom he interacts.

The extent to which others are involved in the initial recognition of problematic experience depends upon the nature of the experience in question. For example, pain and emotional states, though sometimes having external indicators, may not be perceived by others until alerted by a verbal statement on the part of the individual concerned. In these cases their participation is invited by the sufferer in the form of a complaint. Conversely, where changes in the structure or function of the body or the person are externally observable to others then it may be they, rather than the person involved, who trigger off interpretive activity by claiming that something is wrong.[1] As Dingwall has suggested, this 'mutual monitoring of health status is an integral part of the general mutual monitoring of interactional competence in any social interaction' (1976:99).

In the remainder of this chapter I will refer to the problematic experiences that give rise to and are ordered by interpretive activity as cues. In his study of children with poliomyelitis, Davis (1963) uses the concept of cue to describe some of the interpretive processes via which a diagnosis was eventually made. The children who were subsequently identified as polio victims initially complained of minor symptoms such as sore throat, stomach ache, or fatigue. These complaints were attributed by the parents to common childhood ailments, minor mishaps, or malingering. The concept of cue refers to those events which challenged this initial perception of the child's problem and led to its revision. Here, I will use the notion of cue to look at an earlier stage of the interpretive process: the initial recognition of some departure from a state conceived of as normal, usual, or routine. These cues, by disturbing the taken-for-granted sense of order and the unnoticed everyday functioning of the body and the person, alert the sufferer and those around him to the possibility of such a departure.

The women I interviewed described three types of cue that gave rise to the suspicion that something might be wrong. I have called these symptomatological, behavioural, and communicative cues.[2] Symptomatological cues involve changes in physical or psychological states that are experienced by the individual concerned or observed in another. Typically, they involve some change in the way one feels or some change in external appearance. Behavioural cues refer to observed changes in behaviour or conduct on the part of another, and communicative cues consist of claims made by an individual to others or others to an individual that all is not as it should be. I refer to these entities as cues rather than signs and symptoms since they are only constituted as signs and symptoms when they are interpreted as the indicators of an underlying organic or psychological problem. As some of the data extracts I discuss later will reveal, these cues can and were often seen to have their origins elsewhere. That is, they were taken to signify other categories of event.

Symptomatological cues which pertain to the physical or psychological condition of an individual may be experienced by the sufferer as a change in the way he feels:

(G1) (Mrs G) 'If something hurt me or if I felt just perhaps shattered, tired or headache, something like that then I'd wonder what was wrong.'

As far as others are concerned, symptomatological cues usually involve some change in external appearance. Mrs G talking about her husband:

(G2) (Mrs G) 'I would worry if I felt he looked tired in his facial expression, if he looked pale or tired or very flushed so that he looked . . . something like that, or drawn.'

(Int.) 'Why would you worry about those things?'

(Mrs G) 'Well, obviously because there was a change . . . just sort of a fact really isn't it?'

and her baby son:

(G3) (Mrs G) 'The last time I took Daniel to the doctor's he had a really bad, a really high temperature about five o'clock at night he was sat on my knee, been sort of mouldy all day you know, sleeping a lot of the time and he was burning . . . he was just sat on my knee and you could see the glow coming off him, it was really bad so I rang the clinic.'

Changes of this sort indicate that something may be wrong and call for monitoring of the individual concerned or some action to clarify or resolve the suspected disorder:

(S2) (Mrs S) 'Sometimes Michael comes in from school and he's a bit pale, not because there's anything wrong with him but I think it's the journey home sometimes, they don't always sit him properly in his wheelchair, sometimes they tighten him up in his wheelchair, put the strap on and they probably have to keep stopping and starting 'cos they let other children off the coach, he comes in and you know he's as white as a sheet and oh, what's wrong with him you know, you know normally it's only the journey. I usually give him as I say his Junior Disprin, give him a drink . . . I keep coming in and having a look at him and asking if he's OK and then I can see his colour coming back and then I know he's all right.'

For Mrs S, the fact that Michael comes home looking 'pale' or 'white as a sheet' is a potential indicator that something is wrong. As she added subsequently, 'he's a fit boy, he's usually got quite a good colour'. However, she has an explanation at hand which, derived from past experience, enables her to routinize the problem, 'nine times out of ten it's probably because he's had a bad journey home'. Faced with these two alternatives she adopts a wait-and-see strategy and monitors his external appearance until she can see his colour coming back; 'then I know he's all right'. The bad journey home hypothesis is then taken to be confirmed.

Behavioural cues involve some departure from a conception of an individual's normal activity. They constitute noticeable events which indicate, and in turn are explained in terms of, an underlying problem:

(P1)   (Mrs P) 'We feel a bit worried about my father as he seemed a bit on the depressed side, I think, you know, he's gone very sort of quiet so we thought it was a good idea for him to see the doctor perhaps.'

(P2)   (Mrs P) 'Well, Lindsay said it . . . she said she's got this spot under her foot which hurt her and we looked at it and I took her along to the doctor because she came home limping from school. I had noticed it but, you know, I thought well maybe it's just something that's rubbed a little bit, maybe her shoe or her sock, you know, and when she started this limping, well, we'd better see what it is and I took her up to Dr Z.'

In the first example, Mrs P talks about her father who, following increasingly frequent falls, had been persuaded that he could no longer look after himself and moved in with one of his other daughters. Prior to the move I asked Mrs P if she thought he would be happy to leave his own flat. She said, 'Well, this is the problem, one doesn't really know. I'm not too sure whether he will 'cos he does love it round there'. Alert to the fact that his move may create problems, Mrs P and her sister noticed that he had gone quiet, had attributed this to depression, and decided to have the doctor to see him. The second example illustrates how a behavioural cue causes an initial interpretation of a problem to be redefined. When her daughter first complained about a sore spot on her foot Mrs P ascribed it to 'something that's rubbed a little bit, maybe her shoe or her sock'. However, when her daughter came home limping it was seen to be something other than a simple abrasion and a doctor was consulted to 'see what it is'.

Symptomatological and behavioural cues become organized into what may be termed cue inventories. These inventories consist of the typical ways in which given disorders or disorders in general manifest themselves with regard to given individuals. They allow actors to monitor others by providing a range of surface appearances which may be immediately attributed to underlying problems. Inventories may be category-specific, applicable to a category of individuals such as men or children or, more usually, they are person-specific, applicable to particular persons. The former are derived from a socially given stock of knowledge, the latter from personal experience of the individuals in question. For example, the respondents described cues which were typical of the way in which certain problems could be recognized:

(N1)   (Mrs N) 'I know if I'm going to get a cold, I get this feeling at night, you know, that roof of your mouth smarting feeling.'

(S3)   (Int.) 'Do you find it [having a handicapped child] sometimes gets on top of you?'
       (Mrs S) 'Sometimes . . . every so often. I know when I'm going to

be like that because I start feeling all weepy, you know, and I generally feel as if I want to scream. I do sometimes, it does me good.'

(N2) (Mrs N) 'Well, you can generally tell if the girls [her daughters] are out of sorts really . . . if they're kind of mooning around, they don't want to eat, that sort of thing.'

(P3) (Mrs P) 'With Martin if he isn't sort of well he usually wants to be cuddled a lot and he gets a bit listless or something like that.'

These patterns form part of the stock of knowledge at hand which an individual can bring to bear on the situations with which he is faced. They are derived from experience and provide a context in which cues may be situated such that they not only point to the fact that something is wrong they may also suggest a diagnosis. At the second interview I asked Mrs P if there was anything in particular she might notice that would make her think her husband was not well:

(P4) (Mrs P) 'Well, if he began to get unreasonably irritable I would watch that because I think I told you that some, oh a few years back now he did have a bit of a breakdown and he had to have treatment for it and that was one of the things the children couldn't understand why daddy was so irritable, so cross and would shout at them for no apparent reason. I would definitely keep an eye on that. Or if, you know, I occasionally I have noticed him rubbing his chest and I will definitely keep an eye on that because in his younger days he had pneumonia twice so I don't like to . . . if he does get a cold and the cough goes on I will automatically make an appointment for him, you know, because I think that's something that should be watched with him.'

Here, 'unreasonable irritability', 'rubbing his chest', and coughs that 'go on' are seen in terms of Mr P's biography. These cues are taken as potential indicators of past states of affairs that could recur. Hence, the necessity for them to be watched or managed in other ways such as making an appointment to see the doctor. Although medically speaking the episodes of pneumonia and nervous breakdown are closed, that is, the patient was cured, socially speaking they remain open since they have implications for the future and are used in the cognitive organization of the present. Mr P is an ex-pneumonia patient and an ex-case of nervous breakdown and these facts may be taken into account in making judgements about his current health status.

These sign systems, consisting of indicators and an underlying state of affairs to which they point, in conjunction with the observation that what has happened in the past can happen again, allow predictions about the future to be made. If on one occasion an event has been preceded by certain signs then it is assumed that if the event happens again it will be preceded by the same signs. The following extract, taken from my fourth interview with Mrs P, illustrates the expectation that the future can be so predicted and the consequences of a breach of that expectation. Mrs P had just told me that her husband was depressed:

> (P5) (Int.) 'Is he? How does it show itself this depression, I mean . . .'
>   (Mrs P) 'Irritability . . . erm, oh sort of withdrawn a bit in a way, easily gets niggly with the children or things in general, you know.'
>   (Int.) 'Is he much different from his normal self?'
>   (Mrs P) 'Well, perhaps not . . . it's very difficult, when he had the sort of the type of breakdown that he had before I knew it was sort of coming but this time I didn't so that was why it was a double shock in a way when he said about it, erm . . . no, most people wouldn't know a thing was wrong really.'
>   (Int.) 'So did you notice or was it him just mentioned it to you?'
>   (Mrs P) 'Oh, he told me.'

In this extract it is clear that Mrs P anticipated that she would be able to recognize when something was wrong with her husband in much the same way as she had before. In this instance, however, the pattern his biography led her to expect did not appear; last time 'I knew it was sort of coming but this time I didn't'. It was not until he told her he was depressed that she had any idea of what was happening. The sign system that she employs has here broken down, it is inadequate to allow her to make predictions as expected since the underlying disorder has appeared without its customary indicators. It is this breach of her sense of order that gives rise to what she describes as a double shock. First of all, she was shocked that he had become depressed again and second, she was shocked that she had known nothing of it until he had told her.

It was often the case that more than one type of cue was mentioned by the respondents in their descriptions of how they came to realize that something was wrong with themselves or others with whom they interact. Faced with one type of cue an actor may wait for further cues to confirm the initial suspicion that something is wrong. These subsequent cues not only confirm that suspicion, they may point to a diagnostic label or enable a choice between alternative labels to be made.

> (P6) (Mrs P) 'Last Friday Lindsay ran a temperature for no apparent reason. When her father came home from work and I said she's been a bit listless today, I said she's been out playing and she'd been out all day on Thursday playing with some friends around the corner but whenever she came in she just wanted to flop out on the settee. And Friday although she'd been out whenever she came in whether it was for a meal or for a drink or in general in and out you know, she just sort

of flopped on the settee and put a cushion and put her feet up you know and I felt her and she did feel a bit hot and by tea time she looked a bit flushed for her. Colin took her temperature and it was nearly 103 so of course we put her to bed.'

(R1) (Int.) 'How did it [the chicken pox] show on her, did she complain of anything or . . . ?'

(Mrs R) 'She had spots . . . I noticed a few days prior to the spots she wasn't quite herself, she'd lost her appetite and er she was a bit irritable and I was a bit concerned because my husband hasn't been well and I wondered if this was reacting on her. So in fact when the spots came out I was very relieved that it was the reason, so I was quite happy about the chicken pox.'

In the first case a series of cues are assembled over a period of time and give rise to a definition of disorder. Noticing that her daughter had been a bit listless for a couple of days Mrs P mentioned this to her husband who subsequently took her temperature because she felt hot and looked flushed 'for her'. Symptomatological cues were used to elaborate behavioural cues and led to action which revealed that these were indicators of an underlying problem. In the second case Mrs R noticed similar behavioural cues with regard to her daughter and applied a tentative diagnosis. Mr R, who was being treated for depression, had recently spent two weeks as a patient in a psychiatric hospital. Consequently, Mrs R had had to provide her children with an explanation of why their father was going into hospital: 'I haven't wanted to tell them exactly what was wrong because I think that could worry them very much'. Nevertheless, Mrs R remained concerned about how this might affect her children and initially connected her daughter's irritability with her husband's illness, 'I wondered if this was reacting on her'. When the spots appeared, however, this interpretation was revised:

(R2) (Int.) 'Did you know it was chicken pox when the spots came out?'

(Mrs R) 'Yes, yes . . . I checked it with Dr Spock and the description tallied so I phoned Dr M and told him.'

Here, a symptomatological cue not only confirms the definition that something is wrong, it brings about a revision of an earlier depiction by suggesting an alternative diagnosis and leads to action that substantiates that alternative. As Mrs R said a little later in the interview, 'I was pleased when Alison developed spots because it explained her strange behaviour'. I take it that Mrs R was relieved because a diagnosis of chicken pox transformed what might have been a complex problem into a relatively routine childhood illness. I also take it that symptoms such as spots challenged the initial interpretation since it is assumed that problems of that kind would manifest as disorders of behaviour alone and not as changes in physical condition. Moreover, the initial interpretation of the problem presupposes a range of fairly complex assumptions about children and their response to trouble in the family. Some of these I outlined in Chapter 3.

While later developments of this kind confirm definitions that have been tentatively applied or lead to a revision of the diagnostic label employed, they also bring about reinterpretations of earlier events. These events may have been seen to be consistent with a normal order of things or accorded little significance until recast in the light of emerging cues. Here the documentary method is used in reverse whereby an underlying pattern is identified on the basis of one event and used to give meaning to prior events by redefining them as initial indicators of that pattern.

(S4) (Mrs S) 'Talking about Joanna, she was sick. Er, it was just before their Christmas party at the nursery school . . . and erm I'd got all the evening meal ready and she just said I want to go to bed. So I really knew there was something . . .'

(Int.) 'That's unusual is it?'

(Mrs S) 'wrong with her, for Joanna to want to go to bed at . . . well it was five o'clock. And I said alright, we'll take you up to bed sort of thing. She went in, I tucked her up and that . . . er, she didn't tell me what was wrong, she didn't say she felt sick, I just thought she was probably feeling a bit tired, you know . . . once again, neither of them are sickly children, and erm about half past eight she was banging on her door and my husband said he'd go up and he went up and he came straight down and said you'd better come up she's been very sick.'

In this case a child's request to be put to bed is initially ascribed to tiredness until revised following the appearance of a symptomatological cue. As a result of this revision the request becomes reconstituted as a symptom of an underlying disorder.

While symptomatic and behavioural cues may be noticed which are read as indicators that something is wrong, it is frequently the case that nothing amiss is observed until the person concerned communicates some problematic experience to others. This is particularly the case with disorders which may not be directly available to them. Certain subjective experiences such as feeling sick, pain, and a variety of emotional states may not have external manifestations. Though the person concerned may first become aware of the potential problem via a symptomatological cue, it is only via a statement or complaint that the problem is made public. Thus, though as part of the social role to which they orient, mothers are expected to monitor and identify changes in the health status of members of their family, they must frequently rely on problematic experiences being communicated to them.

For example, in data fragment P5 Mrs P knew nothing of her husband's depression until he told her, despite the fact that his biography had led her to expect that certain behavioural cues would alert her to a recurrence of the problem. Since there were no external manifestations of his emotional state a communicative cue was required to alert her to the onset of his depression. Similarly, when Mrs R's daughter caught chicken pox it was reasonable for Mrs R to expect that her son would get it as well. The first indicator that he did have it was when 'he just said he didn't feel well'. This was confirmed later when a symptomatological cue, 'spots', appeared. In this case the communicative cue was elaborated by the symptomatological cue and both elaborated by their context so that they not only indicated that there was a problem but pointed to a specific diagnosis. Occurring within a household where one member had already succumbed to a virus infection the cues confirm the expectation that other vulnerable members of the family would catch it as well. Where communicative cues are the first indication that something is wrong with an individual, they may be seen in context or elaborated by a search for other cues which confirm the original interpretation and, in some cases, allow a lay diagnosis to be made.

In addition, there is an expectation on the part of the women I interviewed that sufferers will use communicative cues to indicate to others that some departure from normal exists. In the following extracts the respondents readily assert that these cues were used routinely by members of their families:

(G4) (Int.) 'Do you think your husband gets anything he doesn't bother complaining to you about?'

(Mrs G) 'No, I don't think so . . . he'd let me know, yes, definitely.'

(Int.) 'Even though it was something he wouldn't bother going to the doctor with?'

(Mrs G) 'Yes, yes, he'd tell me. Well, he usually tells me . . . more than likely he tells me about six times a day.'

(F1) (Mrs F) 'If he [Mr F] isn't well I think he would say. Sometimes he comes home and says, "I've got a sick headache today", which is usually following some big meeting he's had at work, he's had to do a lot of talking and, you know, probably sort of worrying about the job gives him a bit of a headache . . . he always tells me.'

(S5) (Mrs S) 'Oh, Mike [her husband] never complains. If he did . . . you know, he's like most men, if there's anything wrong he'll have a moan about it but, you know, he doesn't really have anything wrong.'

(R3) (Mrs R) 'I think whenever the children have not been well they have complained.'

What past experience has shown to be routine or usual is often used to anticipate what will happen in the future. Any breach of the expectations based on past experience becomes a noticeable event that may call for an explanation. Alternatively, as shown by the next two extracts, these events may be characterized as strange or funny:

(P7) (Mrs P) 'Since I last saw you I have had Martin to the doctor, he did have a mild dose of tonsillitis, about the same time as Lindsay had her chest and throat infections so I presume the germ sort of passed on a bit really, but, er, he had just a shortish course of antibiotics and . . . he wasn't ill with it, he just said one morning you know that . . . he hadn't told me this was the strange thing, he'd got this cough and cold and as I was taking Lindsay to the doctor, I thought well I'll ask him as well. And he said to the doctor, my throat's sore, he didn't tell me this and I didn't know, I hadn't a clue, he hadn't complained about it and the doctor looked and he could see there was a bit of inflammation there and the tonsils infected. So, of course, he gave him a course of antibiotics. It quickly cleared him up with no bother at all.'

(S6) (Int.) 'Anything wrong with the children over the last two or three weeks?'
      (Mrs S) 'No, apart from Joanna being bitten by a little boy at nursery school. She came home not long ago with big bites on her shoulder, really nasty ones they were. But the funny thing was she never complained, she didn't, you know . . . in fact she was quite upset when I told her she musn't let him bite her.'

In both of these cases there is an expectation that the problems described would be mentioned. This expectation also means that in the absence of a complaint it may be reasonably assumed that nothing is wrong. This connection between no complaint and nothing wrong is implicit in S5 above. As Mrs S says of her husband, if there's anything wrong he will complain but he never complains because he never really has anything wrong. Given this assumption, an actor cannot be held responsible for taking no action with regard to a sufferer who has not communicated a problematic experience. For example, Mrs F's mother 'suddenly had a very bad time' with her arthritis and was in such pain that she slept in a chair for two nights without telling anybody:

(F2) (Int.) 'She, she didn't phone you, she told you about this when you went to see her did she?'
      (Mrs F) 'Well, the next-door neighbour 'phoned me up and told

me, did you know, you know aggressively, did you know your mother hasn't been to bed for two nights? I mean, I don't know if she doesn't tell me, I'm always 'phoning her up. Anyway . . . so . . . no, she hadn't told me personally so I had to make out the neighbour hadn't 'phoned me otherwise it would have looked as though we're spying on her, you see.'

In this extract Mrs F invokes the assumption that all may be taken to be in order in the absence of a complaint to defeat a potential charge of neglect. Mrs F cannot be held responsible for not doing anything about her mother since she cannot possibly know that something is wrong if she is not told. Moreover, she presents her mother with adequate opportunities for communicating any problems she might have, 'I'm always 'phoning her up', in which case it is her mother who is to be seen to be at fault. As Mrs F said later in the interview, 'she slept in a chair for two nights without telling anybody, silly old dear'. Once she did know that her mother was in severe pain she arranged for a doctor to visit her at home. A similar rationale is presented by Mrs S in extract S4. When her three-year-old daughter asked to be put to bed at five o'clock Mrs S 'knew there was something wrong' but initially interpreted the request as a sign that 'she was feeling a bit tired'. Though she was subsequently 'very sick' the initial interpretation is justified by the fact that 'she didn't tell me what was wrong, she didn't say she felt sick'. There was then no cue which would allow Mrs S to anticipate what would happen and, as a consequence, nothing on which to base preventive action.[3]

Such is the importance of communicative cues that communicative incompetence poses problems for the recognition of disorder. Communicative cues may be required to recognize disorder *per se* or to elaborate symptomatological or behavioural cues so that judgements about the type or nature of the disorder may be made. In the absence of communicative competence, communicative cues are not readily available, the assumption that no complaint means that nothing is wrong is suspended and strategies adopted to acquire information which would usually be provided by the sufferer in the form of a complaint. Mrs S's son, Michael, for example, was brain-damaged and unable to talk:

· (S7) (Mrs S) 'With Michael he's very special, I mean, you know, he can't tell you when he's in pain unless I ask him different questions all about different parts of the body.'

As reported above, Michael sometimes came home from school looking 'a bit pale' or as 'white as a sheet' which led Mrs S to suspect that something might be wrong:

(S8) (Mrs S) '. . . but then I say to him, is anything hurting you, Michael, you know, I go through all the different things and I just give him a Junior Disprin to be on the safe side.'

Mrs S was very attentive to Michael and constantly on the lookout for indications that all might not be well. She had taught him to nod or shake his head in response to her questions about different parts of his body. During the time I interviewed her she was particularly concerned about his left hip, which had been operated on some nine months previously to give him greater mobility. Since the success of the operation could only be determined in the long term, she was constantly looking for signs, such as pain, which would tell her that he was not progressing as he should be. Whenever she noticed him looking a bit pale or if he drew his breath when she lifted him from his wheelchair, her first question was always 'Does your leg hurt, Michael?' Because he could not readily provide her with that information he was monitored closely and action taken 'just to be on the safe side'.

Michael represents a more extreme version of a problem that may be encountered with other non-components, such as children, in general. Though children who can talk may be able to indicate verbally when they are in pain they may be seen to be incapable of giving descriptions of subjective experiences which would allow those responsible for them to make judgements about the type and nature of the problem:

(P8) (Int.) 'Erm . . . one night Martin [respondent's six-year-old son] woke up with pains in his legs, didn't he?'
(Mrs P) 'Yes, that's right, yes, yes . . . he does get this just now and again. I wonder really whether it is just a form of cramp, 'cos when they're little like that they can't really explain fully to you and he says, oh it's all in my legs.'

Because Martin was only able to give Mrs P a vague description of his pain she was unable to decide what the problem might be. Mr P claimed that he was suffering from growing pains, a category of disorder that Mrs P did not accept. She suspected cramp, but was not altogether sure of that as a diagnosis since her son was too young to provide a more specific account. In the end she said 'I just don't know really'. Because the pains in his legs happened infrequently she had not taken him to the doctor for a professional opinion.

Each of the three types of cue may be elaborated by the others or, as I have indicated, may be elaborated by context. There are two types of context which are used in this way, biographical and time-place contexts. Both consist of a given body of knowledge, concerning a specific individual or a given time and place, which may be employed in providing depictions of cues and tentative diagnostic labels. Such contextual elaboration is of particular importance with respect to behavioural and communicative cues. Because it is assumed that we have control over what we say and what we do and can direct this to our own ends, behavioural and communicative cues may be seen in terms of the motives of the person concerned and subject to a variety of discrediting interpretations. By contrast, symptomatological cues, to the extent that they are externally observable, are their own verification.

In the following extracts, both taken from interviews with Mrs S, biographical and time-place contexts are invoked in her attempts to make sense of various observations with regard to her daughter:

(S9) (Mrs S) 'Well, with Joanna, I think I might have mentioned it before, she gets very flush, her face goes bright red and er she says "I'm tired, I want to lay down", and she lays down on the settee and she'll go off to sleep. And then I do worry because, well, erm, in fact I know now the doctor says she's got funny tonsils . . . he said that her tonsils were a little bit funny and she might every so often have a little bit of trouble and we'll see what we're going to do about them a little later on when she's older.'

(S10) (Mrs S) 'I keep thinking that she's going to get something 'cos at nursery school every child has practically got mumps, chicken pox or some measles or tonsillitis at the moment. You know, you go up there and there's three off with mumps today, you know, and another with tonsillitis, there's chicken pox and measles, but so far she seems to have kept free of it.'
(Int.) 'You've not noticed any signs or anything?'
(Mrs S) 'Well, this morning at nursery school I thought she was a bit pale and, erm, a couple of times she looked a little bit weepy but the first time was because they forgot to give her a biscuit 'cos it's not her regular morning and her name's not on the register, and, erm, I thought it might be to do with, you know, at first because there's so many things round . . . there was two or three children a bit nittery about different things so we all thought oh they're going to be down with something.'

In the first case a variety of cues are situated within Joanna's biography as a child with 'funny tonsils' to become potential indicators of trouble with her throat. Her biography, like that of Mr P referred to earlier, indicates a weak spot that may be expected to be bothersome from time to time. In the second example, cues are seen within a time-place context of 'there's so many things round' to construct possible depictions of those cues. In this particular instance an alternative explanation was found to account for these which indicated that, for the moment at least, Joanna was free from disorder. However, the time-place context establishes the possibility that Joanna will get something; consequently, any definition applied is for the here and now only and monitoring action is called for to locate symptomatological cues that may yet appear:

> (S11) (Mrs S) 'I've been feeling around here [indicates Joanna's neck, Joanna being present at the interview] and I've looked at her back and tummy and chest but there's no spots or lumps yet, but it'll take a bit of time to come up.'

The cues identified by the respondents as indicative of underlying organic or psychological problems are culturally relative and socially sanctionable. That is, they are part of a culturally-determined sign system that members are expected to employ in recognizing that all is not well. Consequently, individuals may be held responsible if these cues are not interpreted adequately. Parents in particular are expected to know when their children are not well and to take action accordingly. Hence the necessity to provide justifications when the signs and symptoms of disorder are not initially seen to be such. Conversely, they are also expected not to interpret 'normal variation' as the signs and symptoms of underlying problems. Burton (1975) has indicated the negative labels that may be attached to mothers who present as problematic babies falling within particular doctors' definitions of normal development. Similarly, doctors' complaints that a large part of their time is taken up with consultations which are inappropriate or for trivial reasons (Cartwright 1967; Mechanic 1974; Gough 1977) are based on notions of what constitutes adequate cognitive and practical activity. In this way doctors are involved in maintaining a particular version of the world by discrediting or substituting their own constructs for the constructs of the patients who consult them.

Explaining disorder: the location of cause and reason

Symptomatological, behavioural, and communicative cues both point to and are explained by a definition of disorder. Achieving a sense of order also requires that the onset of the disorder is itself explained. In some cases such an explanation contributes to the construction of a diagnosis or allows a choice between alternative diagnoses to be made, while in others it is located following a diagnosis. The former involved a search for causes, the latter a search for causes and reasons. Beales (1976) notes that much of lay members' talk consists of causal theorizing, which consists of the identification of objects assumed to be independent of human reasoning and their allocation within a causal nexus of cause and caused. The location of causes and reasons is part of this ubiquitous causal theorizing in which one object or event is seen to precede and be responsible for another object or event. The different between causes and reasons is this: a disease such as polio may be explained in medical terms by a virus which invades the body and damages the nerve pathways responsible for motor function. Lay versions of this might not look very different from the professional explanation. In fact, 'it's a virus' was often invoked by the respondents to account for disorders of various kinds. However, actors may also ask a different type of question requiring a different type of explanation. That is, 'Why has this happened?' Recurrent tonsillitis in a child may be known to be caused by an infective agent but may also be accounted for in terms of a familial trait or features of the environment which predispose the child to infection. A variant of this question, which seems to be asked where the problem is serious or life-threatening, is 'Why has this happened to us?' As the father of one of the polio victims studied by Davis said, 'What is God's purpose in singling out our child for so dreadful a disease?' (Davis 1963:33) and one of Burton's respondents, the mother of a child with cystic fibrosis, asked 'What have I done to deserve this?' (Burton 1975:41). Davis, using a stage conception, referred to the seeking of answers to these questions as the inventory stage, a post diagnostic attempt to make sense of events. This was achieved via a process of redefinition, re-evaluation, and retrospective reconstruction during which the past was realigned to fit the present.

In this study respondents generally constructed explanations to answer the first two questions only; 'Why has this happened to us?' did not appear as the basis for the construction of explanatory accounts. This may be because most of the problems I discussed with my respondents were defined by them as trivial rather than the catastrophe presented by a child with polio. Voysey (1975), however, also noted that this was a question that her respondents, mothers of disabled children, failed to ask. The questions that arise in attempting to make sense of events presuppose a world view just as much as the answers that may be provided. Where serious illness is interpreted as punishment for moral fault then 'What have I done to deserve this?' is a relevant question, just as God's purpose may be questioned if the world is seen as a product of the purposes of a Higher Being. Consequently, the extent to which phenomena can and therefore need to be explained is influenced by the assumptions one makes about those phenomena in the first place.

In this section I explore in some detail the way in which the respondents constructed explanations of the disorders they, or those around them, experienced. I will proceed by examining the features of one case and expanding each point by reference to other data. The case I will consider first is that of Mrs S and her breathing problem, some aspects of which I presented at the beginning of the chapter:

(S12) (Int.) 'Can you remember when you first noticed this shortness of breath?'
(Mrs S) 'I think it was er . . . the beginning of November . . . I

just suddenly, you know, I just couldn't take a deep breath. I thought at first, I thought it was 'cos I always, I mean I'm always rushing around, you know, I don't have much time for sitting down, you know, dashing here, there and everywhere. I do seem to do a lot of things, you know, and when that happened I thought at first that this is what it was, you know, just rushing round. And then I thought well maybe it's because it's too warm . . . we've got central heating but it's not because of that, you know, I'm too warm sort of thing, and erm . . . opening all the windows to get some fresh air, you know, ridiculous. But erm, when it got really bad I thought well, I must go to the doctor and I think I had it a couple of weeks before I went up there. It just suddenly came, you know, one minute I was perfectly all right and the next minute I couldn't breathe.'

(Int.) 'There was nothing that happened that you thought might have brought it on was there?'

(Mrs S) 'Not specifically, no, this is it, you know, now if I ever get these various things, I mean sometimes I get it that I can't sleep and I lay there worrying about different things and it's so stupid because really and truly there's nothing specific apart from when my little boy has to have anything done. I mean he's had this operation and every time he had to go back to the hospital or anything like that then I did get worked up about that, you know, but er . . . there was nothing particular at that particular, you know, at this time, you know, I hadn't to go with Michael for any appointment so . . . It always seemed to start when I was getting the washing machine out and I used to hang over that washing machine and, you know, just kind of gasp for breath. And I still do. I've done the washing this morning and it's just the strangest thing. I will probably not think about it sometimes and then as soon as I've got the washing machine I suddenly start taking deep breaths. It's the strangest thing. Whether it's just coincidence or what I don't know or just psychological.'

This extract immediately followed that presented in S1 in which Mrs S described how she had seen her doctor about her problem and had it diagnosed as 'nerves'. This allowed her to construct a causal pathway linking her situation as the mother of a handicapped child with this and other disorders. As I shall describe in more detail later, this involved positing 'worry' and 'nerves' as intervening variables. Here, Mrs S gives some indication of other causes she claims to have considered prior to consulting the doctor. This illustrates what is a common feature of the construction of explanations. Various causal mechanisms may be identified as potentially responsible for an object or event. Subsequently, evidence may be assembled to allow a choice between these alternatives to be made, and licensed problem-solvers may be canvassed to confirm the choice or be given the responsibility for making the choice in the first place. Mrs S rejected what she initially identified as probable causes on the basis of her doctor's definition. Had she rejected that choice, as some of the women I interviewed did on some occasions, then she would have assembled evidence to demonstrate the superiority of her own choice and discredit the professional construction of the situation.

The factors that Mrs S invokes as potential causes of her breathing problem are chosen from a range that are available within a particular culture. Moreover, those that are considered on any given occasion are probably influenced by the nature of the problem to be explained. That is, a culture will not only recognize certain phenomena as causal agents while rejecting others, it also specifies sets of causal nexus in which objects and events are linked together as cause and effect. Consequently, Mrs S is unlikely to identify witchcraft as the cause of her breathing problem since that is not recognized as an entity in the real world in modern cosmologies. She is also unlikely to invoke 'a virus' as the cause of shortness of breath since viruses are not expected to exist in a cause-effect relationship. Rather, she identifies such factors as her life-style, 'I'm always rushing around', or her environment, 'maybe it's because I'm too warm', as possible causes, although these are subsequently rejected. The explanation couched in terms of the environment does seem to have been considered sufficiently plausible for Mrs S to have acted upon it, 'opening all the windows to get some fresh air, you know', though at the time of the exchange she characterized this as ridiculous. Different causes are invoked to account for the 'strange' connection between Mrs S's breathing difficulties and her getting the washing machine out. This, I think, substantiates the point I have just made. Mrs S does not attempt to account for this observation by referring to life-style or environment since it is difficult to see how they could act as causal agents. Commonsense knowledge is inadequate to allow a pathway to be constructed between these factors as causes and the observation as effect. The observed connection between the onset of her breathing problem and getting out the washing machine is so bizarre that Mrs S is not really able to account for it. Two tentative explanations are advanced however. One is 'coincidence', in which two events may occur together but are not connected in any way, the other is 'psychological'. The latter does constitute an explanation whereas the former explains away and renders an explanation unnecessary. No attempt was made by Mrs S to link this observation with the cause of the overall problem, nerves.

In some cases, new facts which appear may challenge an explanation and call for the construction of a new one. In other cases new facts may be seen to support an explanation, as expected if the explanation is valid, or they have to be managed in some way and assimilated into an explanation. Where the new facts do not quite fit, as in this case, judgements about them may be suspended.[4]

Although Mrs S accepts the diagnosis of nerves as the cause of her problem she is not really able to use this to account for the onset of her breathing difficulty. She had learnt from past experience that she suffered with her nerves just prior to an event such as a hospital appointment for her handicapped child. This she attributed to worry about the outcome of these appointments since they were used to monitor her son's progress and report on the success of his recent leg operation. Consequently, she anticipated being 'a nervous wreck' prior to these appointments or 'anything like that' and expected a variety of problems to appear, some of which might require her to consult Dr M. However, she was not able to identify the onset of her breathing problem as preceding or being preceded by an event of this kind. This discrepancy is not taken as a challenge to the diagnosis, rather, as the following data taken from subsequent interviews shows, the facts of the matter are presented in a way to fit the diagnosis:

(S13)   (Int.) 'Er . . . shall we start off talking about your breathing, 'cos that . . . ?'

(Mrs S) 'Er, yes, well that's still with me, sometimes . . . today it hasn't been so bad but, er, yesterday it wasn't too good . . . it's odd this, you know, some days I don't feel too bad, I mean most days I feel fine but I think I probably worry more one day than another day about what's going to happen the following day, you know, or something like that and I think this is when my breathing starts getting bad. It's definitely nerves.'

(S14)   (Int.) 'Do you think there's anything you can do for it?'

(Mrs S) 'Well, apart from going up there again and getting some more tablets I don't think so, I think it's mainly me, I think if I can, which is very hard to, is to stop worrying as such but I think it's subconsciously you do worry. I mean, as I've said before, I think erm, probably Michael, although really and truly he's not as bad as probably, you know, but I suppose it's there all the time, you just can't forget you've got a handicapped child and although he's doing quite well he's doing a lot better than he ever did do, there's still the future. I think that's mainly the cause of it because I don't really worry about much else you know.'

In the first extract the intermittent character of her breathing problem is presented by Mrs S as a product of the intermittent character of her worrying. Her breathing is worse on some days than on others, therefore she must worry more on some days than others. The breathing problem is taken to be the surface appearance of an underlying pattern which is assumed to exist and is embodied in the causal connection she has already constructed. Note that Mrs S does not say she worried more on a given day and consequently her breathing problem was particularly bad, rather she assumes that she must worry more on some days than others because that is what the fluctuating nature of her problem indicates. The conclusion is derived from her theorizing on the topic and not from empirical observation. The main point, however, is that the facts are presented in a way that fits the pre-existent explanation and as a consequence reinforce that explanation.

In the second extract Mrs S makes statements about the nature of her worrying which allow her to continue to present it as a cause in the face of evidence which might reasonably be taken to indicate that it was not responsible for her difficulty in breathing. As I mentioned earlier, Mrs S was not able to locate the kind of incident which usually caused her to worry to account for the onset of her respiratory problem and in this extract she states that she does not worry all the time, 'I mean I'm not worrying as such'. Consequently, in order to continue to present this as the cause of her difficulty which is present all the time, it is relegated to her subconscious, 'it's subconsciously you do worry'. Her situation as the mother of a handicapped child is, moreover, a source of continual stress, 'it's there all the time, you just can't forget you've got a handicapped child'. Aspects of the theory Mrs S employs to make sense of these events are elaborated so that the explanation continues to fit.

Types of cause

Seven different types of cause were mentioned by the women I interviewed to account for their own problems or those of others around them. These I will call environmental, noxious agent, biographical, person type, psychological states, familial, and esoteric. Explanations were frequently constructed from more than one type of cause, or several causes were assembled into a sequence consisting of cause, effect and intervening variables.

Explanations invoking environmental causes can be found in the following examples:

(G5) (Int.) 'I've had a look at some of the things you put in your diary and I'm going to ask you about some of them. Er . . . now about these ulcers, do you get them very often?'

(Mrs G) 'No, only when I go up to Derbyshire. I think it might be a change of water. I used to get them when I lived in Leeds and I used to go back home to Derbyshire then at weekends, sometimes I got them then. I think it could be a change of water.'

(F3) (Mrs F) 'I get a touch of rheumatism in my arm, but as I say, I don't worry, I ignore it and perhaps it'll go away. I think it's caused from driving with the window down.'

(P9) (Mrs P) 'My daughter at the moment they do seem to think she suffers from a sort of hay fever or allergy . . . they're not too sure . . . as I say, I have been noticing for some time now that she's been getting this cough, it seems whenever there's a wind, a certain direction of wind and again I do notice her eyes seem to be a bit puffy.'

(Int.) 'Did the doctor actually diagnose it as an allergy?'

(Mrs P) 'Well, not definitely, he said and he was a bit streamy, Dr S was himself, he said it's quite he said, that she's like me he said, it is when the weather changes, one day you get it warm and then you get it, the wind gets up and erm I had noticed, you know, that it does seem that when the wind gets up that she'll start coughing or perhaps get a runny nose a bit you know.'

Environmental causes such as those contained above are imputed on the basis of observed changes in an individual's environment preceding a problem of one kind or another. As in P9, this environmental theory of causation may be legitimized during consultation with professionals. Though many of the disorders explained in this way were respiratory or involved pain in joints or bones, many problems were seen to be the result of environmental factors. For example, Mrs P claimed that her daughter's nose bleeds and her own swollen ankles were due to warm weather. However, one of the most common connections to appear in lay talk on these topics is the association between cold and damp weather and problems with the chest or musculo-skeletal system. When Mr P complained of pain down the back of one of his legs, Mrs P said,

'I don't know what it was with his leg trouble, he had been doing some gardening I think and er . . . more often than not, well, I don't think he ever takes anything out to sort of kneel on and if we've had buckets of rain he's kneeling on the damp grass and I know myself I've had my knees play up terribly if you kneel on anything damp for any length of time.'

Explanations such as this may be used to inform actions undertaken to manage the problems to which they refer. Following one bout of chest trouble Mrs P's daughter had been kept at home:

(P10) (Mrs P) 'Yesterday it was so lovely she sat out in the garden a bit, you know, and played around in general. I thought, well, it can't hurt her. And 'erm, she wanted to go out today a bit but it's cooler and it's very damp so I wasn't over keen. 'Cos all I, p'raps it sounds silly, but I don't want her to have a sudden change of temperature and get the cough really bad again.'

When noxious agents are introduced as causes they usually take one of two possible forms, either something that has been ingested or something that has been caught. They tend to be invoked to account for symptoms such as vomiting, diarrhoea, and high temperature. In both instances confirmatory evidence is routinely sought in the form of other cases, either individuals who have eaten the same thing or have been in contact and show the same symptoms. When Mrs P's son, Martin, had tonsillitis following her daughter's chest infection she said, 'I presume the germ sort of passed on a bit really'. Even where individuals have not been in contact, a noxious agent such as a virus may be invoked to account for similar symptoms in which case it is identified as 'something going around'.

Where familial causes figure in the construction of explanations, they may also take one of two forms. Problems may be seen to be the product of particular relationships within the family, or they may be seen to be the product of inherited tendencies. Mrs P, for example, offered an explanation of her husband's depression in terms of the former:

(P11) (Mrs P) 'It's all really to do with, the psychiatrists that he saw said it was childhood, goes right back, you see, he had such an unhappy time, his parents were divorced and when he sort of needed a dad he hadn't got one and then his mother married again but stepfather when he was smaller never had any time for him, it was all his sister 'cos she was the sort of baby of the family and he was er kind of pushed aside and this is the trouble, it kind of something, for some unknown reason, can trigger off all the unhappy memories and he does literally go down and down and then hits rock bottom but, erm, it's all sort of to do with that.'

Mrs R and Mrs G both identified problems which stemmed from a family tendency:

(R4) (Mrs R) 'My son had problems very early on in life, he suffered from tonsillitis very severely from the age of three months, it fizzled out when he was about four, just before we changed to Dr M. In fact, my husband had to have his tonsils out when he was an adult, like my son, you know, it seems to be from there.'

(G6) (Mrs G) 'I've got high blood pressure, but we're all blood pressurey, definitely, my sister, myself and me dad, we've all got high blood pressure.'

Where specific aspects of biographies are invoked as causes, reference may be made to life situations, life events, or life stages. Mrs S, as I have already mentioned, explained her problem with her 'nerves' in terms of her situation as the mother of a handicapped child, and others identified life events as the precursor of psychological problems. Mr R, for example, claimed at an interview with his wife where he was present that his 'normally depressive state' had been 'exacerbated by overwork' to the extent that he required psychiatric treatment. And Mrs R, in a prolonged discussion I had with her about depression, offered life events as causes for cases of depression she knew among her friends and acquaintances:

> (R5) (Mrs R) 'With one woman I know it followed the death of her mother after a little time, she was all right for a bit and it happened after that. That erm which I believe is very frequent, the death of someone and then after a time people get depressed.'
> (Later in the same interview)
> 'I mean there's another woman I know who had a sort of breakdown after her husband ran off with another woman. But then this is almost to be expected, I suppose you've got to react in some way. I mean, not everybody has a breakdown but there must be a reaction.'

As I will describe later, Mrs R did not subscribe to a life-events theory to account for her husband's depression, nor did she entirely agree with his diagnosis that it had been caused by overwork. This is part of the cognitive problem under which she laboured and which I shall describe in the next chapter. Clearly, where life events can be seen to be the origins of a psychiatric problem then they are understandable to the extent that they can be predicted.

Life events are not only invoked to account for psychiatric disorders, they may also be seen as the causes of more mundane conditions. Mrs F suffered from recurrent and often prolonged swelling and irritation of the eyes and eyelids, which had been diagnosed by her doctor as an allergy. However, numerous tests at an allergy clinic had failed to identify any substance which could be causing it. Consequently, each allergic attack led Mrs F to a retrospective examination of events which might have brought her into contact with a potential allergen:

> (F4) (Mrs F) 'I had a very bad do with it just before we went to a dramatic conference at Chester and, you know, I looked dreadful the whole time. Er we decided after talking to someone at the conference, an architect chap, he tied it down for me, he said it's the paint, this particular time it was the paint, 'cos Pete was painting the kitchen and we got this special white paint that never goes yellow and he said . . . and it wasn't until . . . I mean I didn't personally tie it down with that, it was alright while everything was being done, undercoat and so on . . . and I did some top coat as well and funnily enough, I mean now it's been said I can say, oh yes, that must be it because my eyes started stinging as I actually started putting this white stuff on the pipes by the boiler. He said there's something in it and he gave it a name, being in the trade he would know, some chemical in it which obviously I must be allergic to and I'm pretty sure he must be right 'cos

since, you know, the smell has gone and we've finished painting the kitchen, I've been all right. I wouldn't use it again just in case.'

Although Mrs F thought that the special chemical in the paint was responsible for her allergic attack, 'I'm pretty positive that was it this particular time', she thought that she was sensitive to several substances, 'I mean we're not always painting, it can't always be that'. This arose because she was unable to connect the same event with every outbreak of her allergy.

At the same interview, Mrs F was also able to find a life event to explain her younger daughter's 'bad throat'.

(F5) (Mrs F) 'My younger daughter has a bad throat, but I suspect it's because she's been, they've been rehearsing at school an awful lot for this Orpheus, she's singing Venus which really is too high for her. I think it's just strained.'

(Int.) 'And how is she today?'

(Mrs F) 'She thinks she might have a bit of a cold but there's nothing visible so whether it's just sort of nerves or as I say whether the throat because she's been singing all these high notes which are a bit out of her range really.'

(Int.) 'It would be a bit of a disaster for her to have a cold?'

(Mrs F) 'Well, it would, yes, this is it. So whether it's psychological or not I don't know but we'll dose her up until we get her on stage, you know.'

In this case Mrs F rejects her daughter's explanation for the event because there is no observable evidence to support it. She substitutes her own life-events theory which may be connected to the problem in two ways. It may result from the physical strain of singing a role which is too high, or it may be psychological, the product of pre-performance nerves.[5]

Some disorders are seen to be the consequence of the life stages that an individual progressively occupies. Childhood, adolescence, the menopause, and old age were all allocated an aetiological role by the women I interviewed. In so doing they made reference to commonsense conceptions of the typical characteristics of individuals occupying those life stages. Mrs G, in attempting to identify a reason for her son being unwell is aware of such a conception: 'I thought at first it could be teething couldn't it, with a baby. Obviously, everybody puts everything down to teething with a baby, but it could have been.'

A similar conception of problems associated with childhood is involved in the notion of 'growing pains' and the often expressed hope that children will grow out of their problems. For example, Mrs S said 'I feel sure she's growing out of it' when referring to her daughter's frequent colds and Mrs F said, 'I used to get hay fever as a child but I've gradually grown out of that, I don't get it any more'.

Other life stages are also seen to embody weaknesses that may predispose an individual to particular kinds of disorder. Adolescence, for example, is seen as a difficult emotional stage, such that when I mentioned people I had known who had been depressed or prescribed psychotropics in their 'late teens' Mrs R commented, 'Ah, yes, well that's a very vulnerable age, isn't it?' Similarly, the menopause is often taken to be a difficult period in which problems may arise. Consequently, it may be used as a device to explain disorders that appear at that stage of life:

> (G7) (Mrs G) 'My mother used to get . . . oh dear, what did my dad call them . . . lurgy bouts.'
>
> (Int.) 'What?'
>
> (Mrs G) 'Lurgy bouts, well just sort of sickness . . . she used to get them a lot on a Sunday, sort of headache and sickness, whether it was the change that caused it, you know, the menopause.'

Old age is the stage of life at which a wide variety of disorders are experienced and expected. Mrs F said of her mother, 'She's got something to complain about, I mean to say, at eighty-four you expect to get all sorts of things'. And Mrs P, speaking of her eighty-five-year-old father said, 'He's very fit *for his age*' (my emphasis). While general level of health is seen to be age-related, specific problems are also associated with ageing. Though she pronounced him 'very fit', Mrs P's father did have hardening of the arteries in his legs which made walking difficult, 'Well, at his age you've got to expect it really', and he often sounded so wheezy that she had encouraged him to see the doctor about it, 'there again, it's one of the problems of old age, their breathing gets a bit that way, you know'. At a later interview, after he had begun to get muddled and confused, his doctor is reported as saying, 'Oh well, of course, it is to be expected, he is eighty-six'. Ageing may also be used as an explanatory device by the not so old. Mrs P, herself only forty-six, thought an episode of swollen ankles was due to the warm weather although she did also comment, 'I suppose my age has got something to do with it'.

Some explanations locate the origins of disorders within the individual concerned by identifying them as a particular type. The problem is seen as one of their response to events or situations. Mrs S, although having a fairly well-defined biographical explanation of her 'nerves' was able to see how this could be exacerbated by the way in which she reacted to her situation as the mother of a handicapped child. Though she often remarked upon the worry that this caused her she said more than once, 'It's silly really, because there's nothing specific to be worried about'. At one interview she continued, 'I think I do worry needlessly when I think about it. But then I'm like that. You just can't change yourself, can you, I mean if that's the way you are?'

Mrs R, in attempting to make sense of her husband's depression, also indulged in theorizing about the aetiological role of his person type. While he preferred to see his current mental state as the product of hard work, she was more inclined to emphasize that it was his response to the pressure of work that was the important factor. In the following extract Mrs R attempts to assess the contribution made by work and his person type to his problem. She had just described how he was very keyed up about a forthcoming meeting at work:

(R6) (Int.) 'Did he use to worry about this sort of thing before he started getting the depression?'

(Mrs R) 'Yes, but not to that extent. He used to get very keyed up about things, he's always had this tendency to get keyed up about things but of course this has become vastly worse since he got more and more depressed.'

(Int.) 'Obviously his work's very important to him.'

(Mrs R) 'Yes, erm . . . yes, but erm . . . well I, and this is my own personal opinion, I think if you're the kind of person who gets into a state about things you'll always find something to get into a state about, which in fact he has done. I mean, if it hasn't been one thing, it's been another so I think the bit about work is a little bit of an excuse although there is a lot . . . I happen to know from talking to other people who work there, there is a lot of pressure and sometimes it is difficult to cope there. Another friend of ours used to work in the same office and he had a breakdown, a bad breakdown and he was in hospital for two months. Again I don't think that was the reason for the breakdown but it didn't help and since he's left he's very much happier and he's a different person. So I think that the work isn't altogether although I said it's an excuse it is . . . I'm not making sense am I?'

(Int.) 'Well, you think it's contributory?'

(Mrs R) 'Yes, this is what I think. But I know where he works there is a lot of pressure but then of course maybe at other places there is also a lot of pressure, I don't know, I think it's largely a matter of how you react to it, to what's going on around you.'

Mrs R does then see the problem in terms of internal tendencies and individual reactions to situations. This construction led her to a pessimistic view of his prognosis:

(R7) (Mrs R) 'I do have worries and reservations about, you know, will he always be inclined to depression because in fact, er, he says, and I'm sure this is true, that he's been depressed ever since he remembers really without altogether realizing it. This goes back a very long way and, of course, I wonder how far can this be cured if it's of such long standing.'

Mrs R also offered a person-type explanation to account for the fact that her husband lost weight while treated as a psychiatric in-patient: 'he lost a lot of weight in hospital even though he said he was eating but the tendency for him I think under stress will be for him to lose weight whereas I'll put it on under stress, he'll lose it'.

It is not only problems of a psychological nature that may be subject to person-type explanations. Mrs F, because she could not definitely identify the substances to which she was allergic, began to see it in these terms: 'I'm allergic, you know, I'm just one of those people who get allergies and put up with them' (F6).

Tension, stress, depression, and worry are psychological states frequently identified as the causes of certain disorders, either directly or, as in the case of Mrs S, as an intervening factor between some more basic cause and an effect. Mrs R, for example, claimed that her husband's complaints of stomach ache and indigestion were psychosomatic, and invoked a commonsense connection between being nervous and alimentary problems to justify that claim:

(R8) (Mrs R) 'Well, he does complain of stomach ache and indigestion which I'm convinced is psychosomatic, absolutely convinced it is because when he's relaxed he doesn't get it and when he's tense he tends to get indigestion and so forth so I am . . . and, after all, it's one of the first things to be affected if you're nervous.'

One of the most common connections made was that between tension and pain of various sorts. Mrs N attributed her husband's headaches to nervous tension, 'he just gets terribly tied up and knotted that's all, I mean it's just complete tension on his part', and her own and her husband's backaches were similarly explained, 'I have backaches, my husband has backaches, it's from being tense, we're a very tense family'. Both Mrs P and Mrs S said they had headaches from being 'tensed up' and Mrs P found the same cause for the intermittent pain from her duodenal ulcer, 'I find it plagues me if I ever get wound up or worried'. On the last occasion on which it bothered her, 'it was probably the upset of, you know, all his problems and that', referring to her husband's recent confession that he had become depressed. Despite a doctor's diagnosis to the contrary, Mrs F claimed that her mother's 'shakes' was due to worry:

(F7) (Mrs F) 'She calls it the shakes, I've got the shakes you see. It's in one arm. The doctor says it's old age, the muscles get weak. I don't know. I think possibly it's worry's got a lot to do with it. My mother worries so much about anyone in the family it seems to start . . . the fact that she was worried about her sister seemed to start her shakes quite honestly. But then that's just my diagnosis.'

A final category of causes I have, for want of a better label, called esoteric. These are frequently invoked to account for the otherwise inexplicable. Mrs R, for example, asked, following an exchange about someone I knew who had been depressed for a number of years, 'Did anything precipitate it or was it just one of those things?' That is, either a specific causal agent must be located or the event is relegated to that category in which phenomena happen for no apparent reason. The particular entity invoked in this category seems to be related to the severity of the disorder in question. Parents of children with life-threatening or crippling diseases may refer to God's will or purpose, while my respondents, considering less catastrophic disorders, were more likely to accept them as 'one of those things'. Since their impact was only temporary, the need for an explanation was less. Mrs S, whose handicapped son might reasonably be expected to constitute a catastrophe, did refer to fortune when she talked about how fit and well he was: 'We're lucky that Michael is as normal as he ever could be as a brain-damaged child, we're very fortunate, you know.'

Similarly, fortune may be invoked to explain why an unwelcome event, expected to be the consequence of some prior event, did not happen. Mrs P, in answer to my question about her father who only had the use of one leg and had recently had several sudden falls, said, 'Fortunately, he hasn't hurt himself. This has been the thing that's so well miraculous in a way, he hasn't hurt himself at all'. However, even with regard to relatively trivial matters, explanations of this type may be constructed. For example, in the following extract Mrs N invokes a conception of a natural order of things which is not to be tampered with to account for the increased frequency with which her husband caught colds after a course of injections:

(N3) (Mrs N) 'My husband is very susceptible to colds. After all his cold injections. I've stopped him having them now. A waste of time. They'd come up with the flu jabs in his office and I'd say to him you're not having one this time. He had a cold and that was that. But they were more recurring when he was having the jabs. Sometimes you can't interfere with nature, it's got to take its course.'

The choice of alternatives

It is often the case that more than one explanation can be constructed to account for any particular disorder. An individual may select from a variety of causal agents to produce two or more explanatory hypotheses or alternatives may be offered by others, including professional problem-solvers. Where this happens accumulating evidence may be reviewed so that one explanation is seen to be the more likely. In the next extract Mrs G describes what happened following her decision to consult the doctor when she noticed her young son had a high temperature:

(G8) (Mrs G) 'Anyway, I thought he ought to see a doctor so I rang the clinic and he had an appointment at twenty-five past six. By the time we saw the doctor it was seven. By that time he'd been asleep in my arms for about twenty minutes and he'd got his clothes on and it's always hot up there and we got in and undressed him so he could listen to his chest and he'd got a great big red rash all over him and he thought he had measles. So, you know, he gave me penicillin, came back and by the time we got him undressed and ready for bed there was no rash at all. It was just a heat rash, that's all. And that was it.'

(Int.) 'And did you bother giving him the penicillin?'

(Mrs G) 'I did, yes. But it was a virus I'm sure because within . . . I had Nathan [a neighbour's child] that day and within two days he'd got exactly the same thing, but he just got over his within twenty-four hours. And Darren [a friend's child] got it as well and he'd been with us the day before so, you know, it must have been a virus.'

Here, Mrs G challenges the doctor's explanation of her son's high temperature, his diagnosis of measles, and presents facts to substantiate her alternative. The doctor's diagnosis rests upon the observations of a red rash. Mrs G is able to demonstrate that this is not a symptomatological cue indicative of an underlying disorder, but the product of temporary environmental circumstances. Her depiction of the rash as a heat rash unconnected with the problem for which she had consulted the doctor is based upon the fact that conditions which might create a heat rash were present and the rash disappeared following a change of environment. The assumption is that a rash due to measles would not have disappeared in this manner. The doctor is therefore depicted as misreading the facts although no criticism is necessarily implied because at the time the diagnosis was made he had no way of knowing of later developments which point to a different interpretation. This disposal of the professional definition of the situation is substantiated by her presentation of a feasible alternative; that is, the high temperature was due to a virus. This is indicated by facts of which Mrs G subsequently became aware. Since two children who had recently been in contact with her son developed the same symptoms, 'sort of tiredness and this really high temperature', a theory of contagion is invoked and a causal agent identified which is known to be contagious.

Discrediting one explanation of events does not always require the elaborate theorizing that is a feature of the above case. Mrs P, for example, simply rejected her husband's characterization of the pains in her son's legs as growing pains by denying the existence of such an entity, 'That's ridiculous, there's no such thing'. In other cases, two explanations were constructed without a choice between them being made. This usually occurred when the problem resolved itself, a common outcome of many trivial disorders which are self-limiting. The problem does not then constitute an imposed relevance, it is transformed from a practical problem into a theoretical one. Unless preventive action is to be a consequence of the experience, two causal theories can be entertained simultaneously.

Diagnosis as outcome of the explanatory process

The above case illustrates another feature of the construction of an explanation of disorder. That is, the labelling of a disorder, its diagnosis, is the outcome of the way in which that disorder is explained. As Mrs G put it, 'You get diarrhoea and sickness with a lot of things, don't you?' Though diarrhoea and sickness may always be taken as indicative of disorder, interpretive work is necessary to determine the specific disorder they signify.

The following extract reinforces the view that lay diagnoses depend upon the location of a cause for any disorder under scrutiny. It also shows how lay diagnoses are not based solely on signs and symptoms but derive from a process in which other knowledge is employed to arrive at a decision. Since any sign or symptom may point to more than one diagnosis this other knowledge may be the evidence upon which one rather than another is selected. This extract follows an account in which Mrs S described how her daughter asked to be put to bed one evening and had subsequently been sick:

> (S15) (Int.) 'You don't know what it was that made her sick, do you?'
> (Mrs S) 'I haven't a clue. I tried, you know, how you do to think back now what has she eaten during the day, did she have anything different. As far as I could see she had what she would normally have, what we had as well. So I just don't know what it was. Yet funnily enough I heard two or three children had this afterwards so whether she'd picked something up from nursery school, one of those quick things, because the girl next door, her two little girls had got it. I usually put it down to something they might have just eaten, I mean children aren't terribly fussy are they when they go to school or anything like that, they're not. I mean, she'd gone to nursery school so it's quite possible she might have had something there. I think it was just something going around because so many children had it.'

In this case two diagnoses of the symptom are considered and the final choice is made on the basis of information about aspects of the case other than its overt manifestations. The two diagnoses involve varieties of noxious agent, either 'something she's eaten' or 'something going round'. The facts indicating one or other diagnosis are assessed and a choice made. Although Mrs S had not given her daughter anything unusual to eat or anything that other members of her family had not eaten, it is a possibility that she could have had something at nursery school that had been responsible for her being sick. While this would account for her daughter's symptoms it would not explain why 'so many other children' had had the same complaint. 'I think it was just something going round' thus emerges as the diagnosis because it fits the problem in question and other observations assumed to be connected to it.

The reinterpretation of cause

Extract G8 also illustrates the way in which interpretations are reconstructed following the appearance of new evidence. In fact, judgements about the meaning of events are often suspended under the assumption that there will be future developments pointing to a particular interpretation of those events. Whatever, a new theory is called for which accommodates old and new observations. At my first interview with Mrs N her younger daughter was at home, having left school with what she described as a very bad head. Just prior to my arrival Mr N had telephoned to say that he had a very bad headache and Mrs N, while waiting for him to come home, had got in touch with her doctor:

> (N4) (Int.) 'Why did you decide to telephone the doctor?'
> (Mrs N) 'Well, because I thought to myself, she had it, OK, it was tiredness or a migraine. Now my husband has gone down with it, it must be a virus. So I just thought I'd confirm with one of the doctors that it may be or not.'

Similarly, diagnoses may be revised when new facts appear. Mrs F had taken her mother to the doctor after she developed a tremor in one arm. Mrs F thought it was caused by worry but the doctor said it was due to old age and weakening of the muscles:

> (F8) (Mrs F) 'Even now I wonder whether . . . you see she's a funny old thing, it wasn't until we came home from the doctor's the second time that she said, 'cos the doctor couldn't understand why it's only in one arm you see if it's the old age shakes one assumes it should be . . .'
> (Int.) 'Yes.'
> (Mrs F) 'It wasn't until we got home from the doctor's that she said to me, "'Cos it's since I banged it you know, I gave it a nasty bang". So maybe it's not old age tremors after all, maybe she's actually damaged the muscle or the elbow.'

The information provided by Mrs F's mother is used to construct another diagnosis which will fit the newly emerged facts. At the same time it resolves the discrepancy between the original diagnosis and the facts on which it was based. That the tremor is due to injury rather than old age explains why it affects one arm only.

Selecting the evidence to fit the explanation

In some of the extracts above the respondents were able to reject causal theories offered by others by demonstrating that the explanation did not fit the facts. In some cases, however, explanations may be accepted although some of the facts cannot be accounted for in their terms. For example, Mrs G had recently been to the doctor with her young son who had diarrhoea and vomiting:

> (G9) (Int.) 'And did you find out what was wrong with him?'
>
> (Mrs G) 'Well, the doctor said it was a virus because I went up to when we got the prescription the chemist said you're lucky, you know, I've just got some of this stomach medicine left, he said there'd been a run on it so, you know, it was just something that was about. I think there's been a lot of it this year, you know. I know families who've had it four or five times.'
>
> (Int.) 'Mm . . .'
>
> (Mrs G) 'But we didn't get it. That's funny isn't it?'
>
> (Int.) 'Why?'
>
> (Mrs G) 'Well, you would have imagined if it was a virus we would have got it.'

Although Mrs G accepts that her son's symptoms were due to a virus, the doctor's diagnosis seems to be supported by the chemist's evidence, she is able to note an anomaly in the fact that she and her husband 'didn't get it'. Clearly, this is expected to be the outcome of a virus infection for, as she points out, 'I know families who've had it four or five times'. This, however, does not seriously challenge the interpretation that it was 'just something that was about', rather it is merely characterized as 'funny'.

Evidence that does not fit an accepted explanation may be selectively disregarded. Alternatively, the theory may be elaborated by the introduction of additional information, which removes the anomaly by deeming it irrelevant. In the next extract Mrs R tries to find what it was that caused her to be very sick one night:

> (R9) (Mrs R) 'Well, I suspect but I may be wrong, I took my son out for a treat to the Wimpy bar and we each had . . . well, he hardly touched his but I ate mine. I suspect it was that but there was another lady with me and she ate hers and she was all right 'cos I phoned her up and she was fine so whether it was the Wimpy or whether it was my reaction, I don't like them anyway and perhaps because I don't like them very much, perhaps that's why it didn't agree with me. I couldn't think of any other reason.'

In looking for an explanation of her symptoms Mrs R attempts to locate a causal antecedent and finds one in something that she ate. However, because she assumes that anyone eating the same things should also show the same symptoms, the explanation is rendered suspect by her discovery that the person with her at the time was all right. Her son who was also present does not figure in this theorizing since 'he hardly touched his' and would not be expected to show symptoms as a result. In order to maintain the theory that the food she ate was responsible, the theory is elaborated by the selective presentation of other facts. This modified version can then be seen to apply independently of the health status of the others involved. This new theory still allocates a causal role to the food that was eaten, but Mrs R personalizes the explanation by introducing as an intervener her reaction to it. In this explanation, the food itself is not found to be at fault; this would account for the lack of symptoms in those who ate the same thing. Rather, the fault lies with Mrs R, 'because I don't like them . . . it didn't agree with me'.

This sort of elaboration can also be employed to preserve commonsense conceptions of the typical structure of the world. At one interview Mrs S expressed concern that her daughter suffered recurrent 'bad throats' and she got them more in the summer than the winter. This apparent contradiction of notions of the environmental causes of respiratory disorders is managed by the introduction of information about children and their activities which shows that the environmental connection does hold.

(S16)   (Int.) 'Do you think it's unusual to get these throat infections in the summer?'

(Mrs S) 'I would have thought so, yes. But when you think that children run around with not many clothes on. You know, they run around without shoes on and things like that. I mean Michael can't do that so I often think anything like a summer infection is due to the fact that they are running around, they get hot I think rushing around, they play very hectically, don't they, children, they get a bit hot, I know she does and then probably she gets a bit cool when she's not rushing around and then I think this is the sort of thing when things do happen. That's what I've found with her. With Michael I can't tell 'cos he can't run around. I mean he sits outside but it's not as if he's running around with bare feet and things like that.'

The explanations which individuals offer for the problematic experiences which they and others face must articulate with commonsense ideas about typical causes, typical effects, and the sorts of mechanisms that typically link them. Though the data I have collected is insufficient to be definitive, it does suggest that the commonsense conception of the structure of the world makes available to members a series of routine explanations for a variety of problems that others may legitimately expect them to employ. In some instances these explanations are reinforced by the opinions of those professionals with whom members come into contact. Part of the way in which an individual may demonstrate his competence as a member of a social order is by invoking socially appropriate causes to explain given events. It does not seem likely that anyone would attempt to explain psychological problems or depression in terms of environmental causes such as a change of water or a change in the direction of the wind. Those who do interpret the world in inappropriate ways are likely to be subject to sanctions in the form of derogatory labels, ranging from 'stupid' to 'mentally ill', which challenge their cognitive competence. In this way cognitive activity is subject to normative constraints.

The way in which explanations of disorders are constructed is of broader sociological interest than that of the cognitive ordering of the world for different explanations of events carry different implications. First, the way an event is defined may depend upon the way the event was brought about. The theories that coroners employ to account for sudden deaths, for example, lead those deaths to be characterized as suicide, homicide, or whatever (Atkinson 1978). Second, actors may account for their actions in a given situation or towards a given event in terms of the way that situation or event is characterized and explained (see Chapter 6). Third, the explanatory devices that actors employ not only allow them to assign sense to past and present events, they also mean that the future can be predicted. Moreover, the particular explanatory device used determines the extent to which the present and the future can be controlled. Problems stemming from environmental conditions are more easily avoided than those seen to originate in inherent personal tendencies. Finally, the way in which events are explained has implications for the status of the persons involved. As Coulter (1974:153), discussing McHugh's work, comments, 'poor biographical experiences (as explanations of insanity) are more admissible for ascription to a stranger than to one's own son, daughter, and spouse on the grounds that one's own responsibilities are implicated in the latter cases'. In this context it is easy to see that explaining a child's illness as a product of a virus infection has different implications for the public character of its mother than if it were seen to be the product of malnutrition. Because explanations may be used to impute or deny responsibility they constitute moral judgements. Consequently, locating the cause of disorders provides opportunities for criticizing others, demonstrating their incompetence, or otherwise manipulating definitions of situations in the pursuit of given ends.

The assignation of severity and significance

In the foregoing sections I have given some idea of how lay members recognize disorder and give meaning to that recognition in the way that they seek to explain the problematic experiences to which they are subject. A further important aspect of conferring meaning on those events is assigning them to categories of severity and significance. Talk about these matters frequently contains references to how 'bad' particular symptom episodes have been and in the course of the interviewing the respondents described disorders in such a way, either spontaneously or in response to my questions, that demonstrated their severity and/or significance. In deciding such matters members must draw on a stock of knowledge which they assume to be shared and socially accredited, so that their judgements can be accorded the status of descriptions of the way things really are and not exaggerations or misrepresentations. I make a distinction between severity and significance, since a disorder may not be severe according to medical or lay criteria yet may be seen to be significant in context.

In demonstrating severity and significance members may appeal to features of the disorder itself, its consequences, and/or the contexts in which it occurs. Where respondents' descriptions appealed to features of the disorder itself, reference was almost always made to time. That is, the longer a disorder lasted the more likely it was, in retrospect, to be characterized as 'bad' or severe:

(R10) (Mrs R) 'I've had a very bad cold which lasted for about five or six weeks and it was really very unpleasant.'

Mrs F is describing an allergic episode in which her eyes had been swollen and irritated:

(F9) (Mrs F) 'Well, it has been very bad, I've had it sort of over a month or six weeks.'

In both of these cases no reference was made to any other aspect of the disorder. In the former, the expectation is that reference will be made either to experience or knowledge derived from other sources about the typical course of a cold to see the categorization as warranted. Mrs F, in the latter example, supplied her own standard for judging the severity of the problem. Whenever she talked about her allergy she referred to this temporal dimension. Experience had shown her that the condition usually cleared up within two weeks and any episode that extended beyond this normal period was seen to be correspondingly more severe, although the symptoms themselves were not any different.

Mrs R, in monitoring her husband's psychiatric condition, used this notion of time as a resource to chart his progress:

(R11) (Mrs R) 'By about November he'd got considerably worse, he was getting more and more depressed. His bouts of depression became more frequent and lasting much longer. In fact they were with him most of the time . . . erm . . . the periods in between when he was, for want of a better word, normal, were getting fewer.'

In defining her husband's condition as 'worse' Mrs R refers to the fact that his episodes of depression were becoming more frequent, that is, there were more of them in a given time and were lasting much longer such that he was depressed 'for most of the time'. In many ways this is similar to what Zola (1973) has called temporalizing of symptomatology in his discussions of triggers to the seeking of medical care. That is, where a symptom reoccurs or lasts, its significance may be reassessed and professional advice sought.

Conversely, the assumed connection between time and severity can be used to trivialize problems and depict them as relatively inconsequential:

(G10) (Mrs G talking about her oral ulcers which she has described as trivial.)

(Mrs G) 'They're just little spots on your tongue, that's all, in a couple of days they just go.'

(S17) (Mrs S) 'At the moment I have no problems but, erm, probably in about a month I'll start feeling nervy again.'

(Int.) 'Does it concern you . . . I mean does the fact that you get like this worry you at all?'

(Mrs S) 'No, not really because I know it's not going to last very long.'

(R12) (Mrs R referring to her son and daughter who had both recently recovered from chicken pox.)

(Mrs R) 'His wasn't quite as severe, erm, it was only a couple of days really that it caused any problems.'

On occasions other features are appealed to to provide for judgements about severity. Mrs R described in one interview how she periodically suffered from migraine in which she would have a 'very bad headache' and 'feel sick'. She went on, 'my brother has them but a little bit worse than mine . . . when he gets them he *is* sick and he has felt . . . he gets double vision with his I think'. Thus, the number and type of symptoms associated with a condition may be invoked to compare cases and define one as worse than the other. Mrs F, in discussing her husband's allergy, minimized it in comparison to her own:

'He gets sort of something that is similar to hay fever although he's never had proper hay fever that I've caught, 'cos I've had hay fever really badly, you know. I think it's something in the garden which affects him. If he does gardening that's when he gets it but normally just to go out and have a picnic in a field or something whereas I would have been sneezing my head off, it doesn't take him like that.'

In constructing definitions of severity and significance, the respondents pointed to the consequences of disorders or the actions that had to be undertaken in order to manage them. In talk about pain, a variety of consequences were mentioned such as being woken up at night, crying, or fainting to indicate its intensity:

(S18) (Mrs S) 'I pull muscles quite regularly [lifting Michael in and out of his wheelchair]. I had one go in my stomach here and one go in my back and one in my neck. And, in fact, when I had this tummy muscle one I couldn't stand up. In fact I fainted with the pain it was so bad, that's another thing I've never done in my life before.'

(P12) (Mrs P talking of her son, Martin, who woke up one night with pains in his legs.)

(Mrs P) 'Oh, it's all in my legs, he said and he really cried with it, you know, it was genuine. It wasn't, er, something put on, 'cos as I say, it really woke him up so it must have been pretty intense I should think.'

Mrs R and Mrs G both referred to actions as consequences to indicate the severity of episodes of pain.

(R15) (Int.) 'Do you usually take anything for your migraines?'

(Mrs R) 'Not usually . . . I did this time because my head was so bad I took some pain killers.'

(G11) (Mrs F) 'I had this real sort of bad pain in my stomach and it was just after I'd eaten, you know, it got really bad.'

(Int.) 'How bad was it?'

(Mrs G) 'Well, it got to the state where after I'd had something to eat I'd be lying, you know, I'd have to lie down, you know, the pain would be quite severe.'

Similarly, the way in which a disorder affects usual functioning is to be read as an indicator of its severity. Mrs R described how her husband had been referred by his psychiatrist for group therapy and while waiting for notification to attend his condition had deteriorated.

(R13) (Mrs R) 'He'd been recommended in September and no word came that he could join. Well, by November he'd got considerably worse and then one day he felt he just couldn't go to work, that's all, he just couldn't face work. So I phoned up the hospital and, er, said he had got worse and what about the group therapy and in fact they put him in within a few days. He then went back to work for odd days but he wasn't really coping well and then he just stopped going to work, you know, it had got worse and he just couldn't face work.'

Mrs R then returned to his GP and asked to see the psychiatrist again. After a wait of four weeks he saw the psychiatrist who, on learning that he had not been working, suggested treatment as an in-patient. The following day Mr R was admitted to hospital.

In subsequent interviews Mrs R again made reference to the connection between severity and function to demonstrate how bad other cases of depression that she knew had been:

(R14) (Mrs R) 'She wasn't very bad to begin with, she didn't get to the stage where my husband got to where he just couldn't face work any more and he couldn't face people and he couldn't answer the telephone and this kind of thing.'

As this extract illustrates, the connection can be used to deny the severity of a disorder. At one interview Mrs R had just recovered from an infection in the maxillary sinus which had been causing her some pain. When I asked her if the pain had been severe she said, 'No, just a nagging pain. It was uncomfortable but I was able to carry on as normal'. Consequently, others may be seen to be exaggerating if their claims are not borne out by expected changes in activity.

(F10) (Mrs F) 'My mother has been worried about her sister who is seventy something and lives alone in Harrow. She had a fall, had a bad . . . well the sister called it a bad fall in the bath . . . well, that's all . . . well you know, the big scene, but she would . . . I mean it didn't incapacitate her, she didn't stop *home* or anything, but my mother worries so much about anyone in the family.' (Respondent's emphasis.)

The women I interviewed invoked a variety of contextual matters to substantiate their characterization of the significance of symptom episodes. They frequently made references to age in managing problematic experiences and claimed that a disorder in a child caused more concern and was more likely to lead to remedial action than a similar disorder in an adult. That disorders in young children are to be treated with some degree of urgency because they are in themselves of significance was invoked as a principle by the respondents in dealing with others such as practice receptionists who were seen to be reluctant to grant appointments with the doctor:

(G12) (Mrs G) 'When Daniel had this high temperature I thought he ought to see a doctor so I rang the clinic and she said, "Must he see the doctor tonight?", so I explained that he was only eleven months old and that, yes, I thought he ought to.'

(S19) (Mrs S) 'I mean my friend's got a baby of eighteen months old and she's had awful chest trouble with the baby and she coughs and has a permanent cold and all the rest of it and when she 'phoned the doctor the receptionist said, oh well, you know I'm sorry but we can't fit you in and Pam said, well it is a baby, you know, and they said well all right perhaps we can.'

Symptom episodes may also be situated within the context of a person type. Mrs R described how her mother who has high blood pressure was sitting watching television one evening when her leg 'suddenly swelled up and was exceedingly painful':

(R16) (Mrs R) 'Well, when I saw it the next day it was still a bit swollen but not very much but it had been exceedingly painful. Erm . . . er . . . the kind of person she is then if she says its exceedingly painful then it really is because she's not one to complain, she'll always minimize everything.'

(R17) (Mr R, who was present at one of the interviews with his wife, was talking about his daughter who had recurrent lower abdominal pain.)

(Mr R) 'It actually was quite nasty, she was in quite a lot of pain with it. She would try and throw herself all over the place and she's not too much of a fusspot in that direction, is she?'

Here, typifications of individuals are used to show that their response to pain can be taken as a valid indicator of its severity since it rules out the possibility that they are exaggerating, lying, or otherwise misrepresenting the experience. At a subsequent interview, I discussed the latter case again with Mrs R. She had taken the child to the doctor who had been unable to find any cause for the pain and had decided not to refer her for further examination. When I asked Mrs R if she thought it was serious, she offered the professional definition, 'Well, the doctor couldn't find anything', to indicate that it probably was not.

Time-place contexts may also be used to situate symptom episodes and accord them a degree of significance. Mrs G had a fairly long history of tonsillitis and throat infections and to indicate her susceptibility to this problem said, 'But even when I was living in Bahrain I had to go to the American Mission for stuff for it there, in that climate, you know'. This derives its force from the assumption that certain problems do not ordinarily appear in certain climatic or seasonal conditions; hence the fact that summer colds usually receive special mention in everyday discourse. Mrs S also mentioned seasonal factors as the reason why she was worried when her daughter went through a period of refusing to eat:

(S20) (Mrs S) 'Joanna went through this dreadful stage of not eating, she wouldn't you know, bits and pieces and that sort of thing but she would not sit down and eat a proper meal. That was a worry to me.'
(Int.) 'Did it go on for a particularly long period?'
(Mrs S) 'A couple of months . . . through the winter time which, of course, made it worse.'

Mrs S often spoke of her belief that eating well and eating the right kind of food was essential to good health. She thought that the success of her handicapped son's hip operation was due to the fact that 'he eats like a horse'. Others whose operation had been a failure showed the tongue-thrusting characteristic of some brain-damaged children with consequent difficulties in eating. As a result, they were weak and frail in comparison to her son who she described as healthy and strong-boned. In conjunction with the assumption that the winter is a time of increased susceptibility, not eating takes on particular significance.

Finally, disorders may be seen in the context of life interests which make them a matter of concern to one individual whereas to another they may be ignored. Mrs F's eye allergy had significant implications for her life interests which meant that she found it difficult to accept the problem and live with it:

> (F11) (Mrs F) 'I mean, I must wear eye make-up. I know my mother says, oh you don't need to and the rest of it but the crowd I mix with everybody does. I mean, we're doing a show, er, we're doing Lilac Time at the end of May. I mean you can't go on a stage without eye make-up because everybody's got to wear it. It's a big hall so you've got to wear make-up, if my eyes are poorly to start with they're going to get worse if I put all this muck on. I've got to be able to use it or give up my hobby, so it bothers me personally very much more so than someone else who doesn't do that type of thing.'

Similarly, when her daughter developed spots on the face, an apparently trivial problem, Mrs F appealed to her current life interests to account for the fact that she was worried about it, 'But as she's doing modelling at the moment, photographic modelling, she was particularly worried about this and that's why she went to the doctor'. Medically minor problems can take on significance when viewed within a social context. It could be suggested that the interpretive asymmetries involved when doctors complain of patients who present with trivial disorders arise because those disorders are not seen in their proper context. Medical judgements concerning severity and significance are made according to a different set of criteria such that different meanings are imputed to events and actions.

Normal disorders

Some of the data presented in this and the other chapters suggest a commonsense conception of what may be termed normal disorders. Although 'abnormal' they are disorders which are taken to be part of the routine experience of everyday life. As such the concept of normal disorders is distinct from the concept of normalization.

Normalization refers to that process whereby what is perceived as potentially problematic is explained in ways which show it to be normal, typical, or unworthy of further comment. For example, Yarrow and his colleagues (1973) have described how the wives of the psychiatrically ill initially normalized their husbands' apparently bizarre behaviour by seeing it in themselves, in others who were not defined as mentally ill, or as a product of their personality or subculture. In data extract S10 Mrs S normalizes her daughter's behaviour at nursery school by seeing it as the product of particular circumstances, 'they forgot to give her a biscuit', rather than as a symptom of an underlying disorder. Other problems such as tiredness may be normalized by showing that they are normal responses to normal life situations:

(S21)   (Mrs S) 'Well, I'm always dead tired but after a day it's bound to be, you know. I mean, it's nothing to see my husband nodding over the television but, erm, we all do that, I do at the end of a day. I find that life is so hectic there's always plenty to do. As I say, if Mike wants to nod off, fair enough, 'cos I know he's had a busy day. I suppose like everybody else he gets tired.'

Normalization may also be achieved by claiming that a potential problem is normal for a member of a given social category. When Mrs G told me that her son had recently had a very high temperature I asked if she had a thermometer and used it to determine how high his temperature had been.

(G13)   (Mrs G) 'No . . . I haven't got a thermometer, I don't know if it's a good thing really, I mean with a baby the temperature can go up and down constantly you know, you could be panic stricken or something like that.'

In offering this rationale as to why she does not keep a thermometer so she can check her son's temperature Mrs G claims that it is normal for there to be variation in a baby's temperature. Consequently, keeping and using a thermometer could lead to this normal variation being incorrectly interpreted as a symptom with undesirable results, 'you could be panic stricken'. Thus, changes in a baby's temperature are not always pathological but can be a normal feature of an individual in that category.

In contrast, the concept of normal disorders does not involve the idea that certain problematic experiences are in themselves normal, merely that their occurrence in given categories of individuals is. For example, it was common for the respondents to speak of 'normal childhood complaints' or 'children's ailments' to which it is expected all children will be subject. As Mrs S said of her husband, 'He's had no serious illnesses apart from the normal childhood ones'. And Mrs R, during a general discussion of the kind of circumstances in which she would consult a doctor about her children, said:

(R18) (Mrs R) 'I know that I expect the normal childhood illnesses. If they had anything that I didn't recognize as a childhood ailment which was bothering them then I'd take them to the doctor. Yes, I'm sure I would because one doesn't expect children to be ill, not *ill*, other than the childhood things.' (Respondent's emphasis.)

Because these childhood illnesses are normal disorders they are expected and, as a result, do not give rise to a great deal of concern. When Mrs R's two children went down with chicken pox she telephoned the doctor to let him know but did not ask him to visit as 'there was no point'. The same kind of disorders appearing in an adult give rise to greater concern because they are not expected as the routine experience of adulthood. Mr R had had his tonsils removed eight years previously which Mrs R said was 'very unpleasant for an adult' and Mrs P, having told me that mumps had 'been going round', said:

(P13) (Mrs P) ''Cos I feel sorry for a girl friend of mine . . . all three of her children have got it, the baby included and neither her or her husband have had it and I thought, oh my godfathers if you get it now . . . I keep hoping she won't poor thing.'

As well as this general class of phenomena, 'childhood illnesses', specific complaints may also be expected to occur in members of that category:

(S22) (Mrs S) 'I think with children, I mean they are sick at times most of them, my friends often say one of the girls has been sick for a night or something like that, you know, but they're alright the next day.'

(P14) (Mrs P) 'Lindsay had a very bad nose bleed once when we were on holiday and Dr M said, oh, it's nothing really to worry about, some children do. I have a friend over the road and her children get nose bleeds quite a lot in warm weather, apparently they say the membranes in the nose are a bit thin.'

Certain disorders are also seen as normal for individuals at the other end of the age continuum. Mrs F, for example, said of her mother, 'she's got all the aches and pains that go with old age'. Some disorders may also be seen to be typical of members of a given sex category. Mrs G, during a discussion of constipation in pregnancy, claimed that abnormal bowel function was a characteristic of many women:

(G14) (Int.) 'Had you been constipated before you got pregnant?'
         (Mrs G) 'Oh yes, you know, I've asked lots of women about this and I'd say that a fantastic percentage say that they are constipated, they don't want to go to the toilet every day and yet most men seem to, you know, with a man it seems to be a certain, you know, you could almost time it, put it down to a time but with a woman it's not at all.'

Normal disorders are then disorders that are routinized rather than normalized. Because they are routine their occurrence does not have to be specially justified. This routinization may have its basis in common conceptions of what is typical or knowledge of what is typical derived from an individual's own experience. Professional definitions may also be sources of routinization and doctors may deliberately or unwittingly influence patients' conceptions of their problems. During the year in which I interviewed her, Mrs P repeatedly expressed concern about her daughter who seemed to be very susceptible to respiratory infections. At one stage she had been prescribed four courses of antibiotics for bronchitis within a period of five months. Finally, Mrs P had demanded that they 'get to the root of the problem' and had been referred by Dr S to the local General Hospital for blood tests and X-rays. Subsequently, Mrs P said, 'Maybe Lindsay is a bit on the weaker side, you know, in comparison to other children'. However, while waiting for her hospital appointment Mrs P took Lindsay to a national children's hospital for a routine yearly check on a heart murmur discovered at birth:

> (P15) (Mrs P) 'And I told them about the bronchitis and the doctor said, "Tell me someone who hasn't had bronchitis", so I presume the weather we've had this winter has been bad weather for bronchitis.'
> (Int.) 'So you don't think Lindsay's abnormal in that respect?'
> (Mrs P) 'I guess not by what the doctor said.'

The doctor's statement, 'Tell me someone who hasn't had bronchitis' is read by Mrs P as routinizing her daughter's chest infections by indicating that it is a problem common to everyone. Mrs P is then able to supply an explanation which locates the weather as cause and revises her initial conception of her daughter from one of 'a bit on the weaker side' to one of 'not particularly abnormal'. Given this interpretation, bronchitis becomes a normal disorder one might reasonably expect given prevailing climatic conditions.

The concept of normal disorders also encompasses a notion of the form in which disorders appear. In many respects this is similar to Sudnow's concept of normal crimes (Sudnow 1973). This notion was usually employed when some departure from this normal form was noticed. This can be discerned in the following extract in which I had asked Mrs F what might lead her to consult a doctor:

> (F12) (Mrs F) 'Well, say it was a cough, it would depend on the cough.'
> (Int.) 'How do you mean, depend on the cough?'
> (Mrs F) 'Well, if it was just a normal sort of cough that you've experienced before, fair enough, but if it wasn't . . . obviously, if you were spitting blood or anything like that then obviously you would go.'

Given that categories of individuals are expected to present with certain disorders, members may be faced with the problem of deciding when that disorder does signify something other than a routine state of affairs. How do mothers, for example, go about seeing an episode of sickness in a child as something worthy of special attention rather than part of normal experience? The limited data I have would suggest that this is accomplished by appealing to the form the sickness takes. Mrs G had no problem in defining her son as ill and in need of medical attention after he had been sick even though she had told me in an earlier interview that he was sick quite often:

(G15) (Int.) 'When he was ill with his sickness . . . I mean you said he was sick a lot as a baby . . .'
 (Mrs G) 'Yes, but this was violent.'
 (Int.) 'How do you mean?'
 (Mrs G) 'Well, you know, he just pumped it all up . . . it wasn't like a normal . . . a sickness where, you know, sort of like with wind when the sickness comes up, but this was a pump, two or three . . . it was all down Roger [her husband], all over the carry cot, Daniel was covered in it as well.'

The recognition that her son was ill did not depend upon his being sick, rather it was the manner in which he was sick that alerted Mrs G to the fact that all was not well. The way in which he vomited on this occasion constituted such a clear departure from the normal form that the alternative interpretation, that this was a routine case of vomiting, was not entertained. Similarly, Mrs S described a case in which the normal form was breached:

(S23) (Mrs S) 'My friend, she gets bad headaches, at the moment she's got to go to the General Hospital, she's been getting these headaches, apart from her normal headaches she was beginning to feel a bit sick and dizzy at the same time and the doctor at first told her she had a touch of migraine but, anyway, she's got high blood pressure and she's got to go to the hypertension clinic.'

While it is tempting to suggest that the departure from the normal form led to the friend's entry into hospital care, it is perhaps better to restrict this piece of data to an illustration of the use of the idea of a normal form. What it does demonstrate is that there are normal headaches and abnormal headaches. Talking about her own headaches Mrs S said, 'It's not migraine or anything like that, just a straightforward headache'. Categories of individuals such as mothers may expect normal headaches as a consequence of their life situation while abnormal headaches require special attention because they are not part of the routine order of things. In Chapter 6 I show how the normal form in which given problems present is offered as the rationale for their management by recipes that have proved to be effective in the past.

Notes

1. Such interpretative activity need not involve the person concerned. See, for example, Smith (1972).
2. Davis (1963) describes four cues, symptomatological, behavioural, environmental, and authoritative. The last two are not applicable in this context since they presuppose that a definition of disorder has been applied.
3. This point is expanded by means of data in Chapter 5.
4. Atkinson (1978) describes several cases in which coroners characterized deaths as suicides on the basis of evidence concerning the mode and location of death although the 'psychological autopsies' of the persons involved did not reveal a state usually taken to be the antecedent of suicide.
5. Note that the respondent does not say this but assumes that the necessary connections will be filled in by a hearer.

5 The construction of definitions of illness

In Chapter 1 I argued that illness is a social construct constituted by the imputation of meanings to various observed or experienced states of affairs. As such it is analytically, and sometimes empirically, distinct from those biological realities called disease. I also drew a distinction between definitions of illness and definitions of disorder. The implications of these definitions for the person so labelled and those around him are somewhat different. Definitions of illness have consequences for an individual's behaviour and relations with others and involve a change in social status. By contrast, definitions of disorder, although they may result in that problem-solving conduct called illness behaviour, do not necessarily have implications for a person's social status.[1] In this chapter I am mostly concerned with the construction of definitions of illness. As Engel (1960) points out, the identification of someone as ill begins with an initial complaint, either by the sufferer or by others. Here, I examine the interpretive work integral to the formulation of these claims and the grounds employed to support or defeat them. The aim is to say something about 'the cultural resources and inferential procedures involved in any warrantable instance of (illness) ascription' (Coulter 1974:114). The basic theoretical point is that social reality is constituted by the use of these procedures and that language and its categories is the medium through which that reality is created and maintained.

Illness-relevant behaviour

While the theoretical problem of illness as deviance is still the subject of theoretical debate, there is agreement that disease and illness involve some departure from a state considered to be normal or routine. This departure may take a variety of forms. It may consist of a change in the physical structure or appearance of the body such as a lump, ulcer, or loss of colour; or it may be a change in subjective experience such as pain, dizziness, or feeling sick, or its report by another, or it may be a change in activity, mood, or behaviour. All of these may be viewed as problems and subject to interpretation and organization. As the analysis in Chapter 4 revealed, they become endowed with meaning when identified as a member of a given class of phenomena. While any of these may be defined as having their origins in an underlying disorder it is not necessarily the case that those so afflicted will be identified as being ill. Illness involves more than the mere presence of disorder.

During discussions about individuals known to them who were or had been ill, the respondents identified some of the grounds on which definitions of illness were applied. Those grounds frequently contained reference to events I will call illness-relevant behaviours and included such things as staying in bed, staying away from work, seeing the doctor, and the like. I call these 'behaviours' rather than 'actions' since they are only partially organized when described in this way. They only become actions, that is, socially relevant, when some meaning is imputed to them. Staying in bed may be construed in more than one way, as indicative of tiredness, laziness, or illness. Because a number of such alternatives is always possible, interpretive work is necessary to resolve the ambiguity this entails. Mrs G, for example, invoked these behaviours in denying that she had been ill during one of the periods in which she kept a health diary.

(G17) (Int.) 'Now, during the period in which you kept the diary and all these things we've mentioned, would you say that you were ill?'
(Mrs G) 'No.'
(Int.) 'Why not?'
(Mrs G) 'Well, because I . . . I didn't have to stay in bed or anything like that and I didn't have to go and see a doctor.'

This account consists of a denial and an accompanying rationale. What is presupposed by Mrs G in offering this rationale is that having to stay in bed and having to see the doctor are actions typical of people who are ill; moreover, that the absence of these behaviours is sufficient to indicate the irrelevance of illness as a description of a given state of affairs. Commonsense knowledge about the behaviour of people who are ill, assumed by the respondent to be shared by the interviewer, is used to make the connection and construct an adequate definition of the event.

Seeing the doctor and staying in bed are then conceived of as typical courses of action exhibited by people who are ill. They form part of a commonsense construct of how ill people behave. On occasions this construct may be used normatively as a description of how ill people ought to behave. In this instance, however, the construct is not used to prescribe certain forms of behaviour, it is used as an interpretive scheme to characterize events or states of affairs. While Cicourel (1968) would maintain that interpretive procedures are necessary to assign sense to settings so that actors can invoke appropriate norms, it also seems to be the case that settings can be characterized according to whether certain norms are seen to be operative. That is, the presence or absence of behaviour appropriate to the status 'illness' may be used in assigning the category to given events or denying that it is applicable. Though it is not necessarily the case that an actor's reconstructed logic, the procedures employed in the reconstruction of events, is the same as his logic in use, the procedures used to assign sense to settings so that the actor can decide on proper actions (Cicourel 1973), it would seem that illness-relevant behaviours are invoked routinely as an interpretive device and not confined to the reconstruction of events. Observation would indicate that the claim to illness is frequently denied by others on the grounds that the individual in question refuses to see a doctor or modify his normal activities in appropriate ways.

Because illness-relevant behaviours are typical courses of action of those who are ill they may be assumed to be characteristic of anyone occupying that particular status. As the following extracts show, they either figured in respondents' descriptions of illness or were the subject of my questioning about it:

(F14) (Int.) 'You say your husband has been ill?'

(Mrs F) 'He had a very bad cold, not really flu . . . a bad fluey cold and a temperature so he spent two days in bed.'

(R20) (Mrs R had been telling me about her daughter and son both of whom recently had chicken pox.)

(Int.) 'Did you have to keep her in bed at all?'

(Mrs R) 'Erm . . . she stayed in bed one day when she really didn't feel well, but other than that she was at home. She didn't go out of course. In fact the first day she did go out for a nice . . . it was a nice bright day and we took her out for a walk. That evening she had a temperature and the following day she stayed in bed and felt quite miserable.'

(Int.) 'And then your son picked it up?'

(Mrs R) 'Yes.'

(Int.) 'Did he show the same kind of symptoms as the girl?'

(Mrs R) 'Yes, except that his prior to the spots didn't last very long he just said the night before he just said he didn't feel well and so I said you know you can go to bed and I think he went up to have a bath and called down I've got it too, I'm full of spots and he did have and that was it.'

(R21) (Mrs R) 'A friend of mine is ill. I spoke to her this morning, she's got erm . . . she's been ill before, something the matter with her blood, she's very anaemic and she has extremely low blood pressure and apparently the two combined aren't very good. She's been feeling quite ill since before Christmas but when I spoke to her today she said at last she is feeling a bit better, but it's been you know, she's erm as I say before Christmas, it's only now she's beginning to feel better and she's really been quite ill.'

(Int.) 'Has she sort of been in hospital or er . . . has she had to stay in bed?'

(Mrs R) 'Erm no . . . she hasn't had to stay in bed but in fact she has been in bed most of the time because she's been too ill to get up, she's resting at home most of the time. The main thing is she musn't walk because walking lowers her blood pressure, she just walks a very little bit, erm she really does very little, she rests.'

These extracts are taken from parts of interviews where the respondents were asked if they, members of their families or others known to them had been ill. All three contain references to disorders and the behavioural consequences of those disorders. That these consequences are presupposed by the questions I asked to stimulate further talk about the cases is indicative of the fact that the commonsense construct involved is oriented to by both parties to the interaction. That is, the interviewer must use that construct as a resource in formulating sensible questions while the respondent must use it in formulating descriptions.

That behaviours such as staying in bed, not going out, doing very little, and resting are presented as the consequences of underlying disorders is of some importance. As I have suggested, these behaviours may be subject to a variety of interpretations. Illness is only one of many labels that may be applied. Consequently, for a definition of illness to be warranted those behaviours must be seen to be the product of some underlying disorder. The significance of explaining illness-relevant behaviours in this way is such that its origins were often made explicit.

(S25) (Mrs S had just described how her three-year-old daughter had felt unwell one evening and had subsequently been very sick for no apparent reason.)

(Mrs S) 'In fact, it's rather funny, oh it's all coming back to me, you know, I'm terrible, yes, she had it on the Tuesday she had that and the next day as I say I woke up feeling a bit sick myself and erm . . . I wasn't sick at all all day but I felt pretty rough and in the morning Joanna went off to nursery school and I was going to take her up to nursery and then go on to Michael's school where they were having their school concert in the afternoon and erm . . . I couldn't go because I felt so sick and I thought oh I'm going to be ill and all I wanted to do was to lay down. So my friend said to me oh you're silly, while Joanna's at school you want to go and lay down for a little while . . . so I did.'

(R22) (Int.) 'Have you had anything you can remember you haven't been to the doctor with or . . .'

(Mrs R) 'Yes, oh yes. I was terribly sick one night which is quite unusual erm . . . I felt this terrible nausea and just felt absolutely terrible and had to go to bed and I was really very sick and had diarrhoea and felt absolutely awful.'

In both of these cases illness-relevant behaviours are presented as the unavoidable consequences of subjective experience such as feeling 'absolutely awful' and 'pretty rough'. When Mrs R says 'I couldn't go to the concert in the afternoon' and 'all I wanted to do was to lay down . . . so I did' her acts are not to be seen as motivated by desired ends. Rather, they are actions imposed upon her and explained by her subjective state, 'because I felt so sick'. Similarly, when Mrs R says 'I had to go to bed', this is to be read as a direct product of an underlying disorder and not as an act that was motivated by any specific purpose on her part. For both of these women the actions they describe emerge out of and are legitimated by the subjective experiences that stem from an underlying disorder. In turn, these actions verify and indicate the severity of those experiences and warrant the imputation of the definition 'ill'.

The interpretive rule that is involved in the above accounts may be employed in another way. If illness-relevant behaviours are the unavoidable consequence of some disorder then the renunciation of those behaviours by an individual defined as ill may be taken as evidence that the disorder is beginning to resolve. At one interview Mrs N used the rule in this way:

(N6) (Int.) 'Have any of your family been ill recently?'

(Mrs N) 'Yes, my youngest daughter a few weeks back with glandular fever.'

(Int.) 'And it meant staying in bed?'

(Mrs N) 'Oh yes, she wanted to stay in bed . . . they always want to stay in bed, then all of a sudden they want to get up so that's a very good sign.'

Here, wanting to get up is an indicator that behaviour is no longer constrained by the underlying disorder. It is a 'good sign' because it means that the person is beginning to recover. Getting better is not only a biological process in which the body overcomes infection or achieves tissue repair, it is a social process in which normal activity is resumed. Resumption of normal activity was often described by the respondents in demonstrating a return to health. Following the description of the episode presented in R22 Mrs R went on, 'But next morning I was fine and went out'. Similarly, after telling me that Michael had woken up one night with a 'funny tummy' Mrs S said, 'Next day he was a bit sick in the morning erm . . . he was all right the next day and went to school'. In these cases going out and going to school are evidence that things were 'all right'.

Illness-relevant behaviours and the construction of definitions of health

The last data extract above indicates that what I have termed illness-relevant behaviours are not only employed in the construction of definitions of illness but were also employed by the women I interviewed to construct definitions of health. On some occasions this involved not having to see the doctor.

(S26) (Mrs S talking about her husband.)

(Mrs S) 'He is healthy, yes he's very healthy. Always has been. We've been married nearly seventeen years now and I don't think I've . . . I think he's only ever visited Dr M twice. Only time he ever has off work is to take Michael for hospital visits and that sort of thing. He had to take him for his six-monthly check-up, he had a half day then you know.'

(F15) (Int.) 'What about your husband?'

(Mrs F) 'He's very healthy.'

(Int.) 'Very healthy?'

(Mrs F) 'Yes, he hardly ever sees a doctor . . . he was about eight years without ever being on anybody's books when we came from Edgware to here. All he contacted Dr M mainly said please will you take me on because it's got something to do with the children. In fact, he had flu about a month ago and he was so unused to going to a doctor that he hadn't got a clue about the insurance thing or who he sent it to or what sickness pay he was entitled to . . . and he had a couple of days off and you know it was quite complicated to him. He's a very fit man.'

(G18) (Int.) 'What's your husband's health like?'

(Mrs G) 'Roger is very good. He's never seen the doctor in the four years we've lived here.'

Theoretical discussions of the concept of health have often noted that it cannot be taken to mean simply the absence of disease but must include some broader notion of well-being.[2] Nor does the lay perspective define health solely in terms of the absence of disease. In fact, someone may be defined as healthy even though they may from time to time suffer a variety of disorders. Rather, as these extracts demonstrate, health is the absence of illness, which in turn is indicated by the absence of behaviours such as going to the doctor or taking time off work. The underlying assumption is, of course, that someone who was not healthy would have to resort to behaviours of this kind. As Mrs G said of a neighbour's child who was always ill, 'he's always on antibiotics, you know, they say to her up at the clinic are you *the* Mrs so and so, you know, they know her name she's had that many prescriptions'. Consequently, not having to see the doctor over a period of time may be sufficient to indicate that someone is healthy. Even professionals such as doctors were seen by respondents to use this interpretive procedure. For example, at one interview Mrs G described how her son had been sick one afternoon after her doctor's surgery had closed so she phoned him at home:

> (G19) (Mrs G) 'He [the doctor] said to me, "Mm, have I seen this baby before?", so I said, "Yes, once at a three-month check-up", by this time he was eight months old and that was the first time you know that he'd ever been ill and I'd rung the doctor and he said to me,"Mm, been remarkably healthy up to now then".'

On other occasions the respondents supported their characterization that someone was well by pointing to the maintenance of normal activity. For example, Mrs S said of her children, 'They've both been very fit, in fact neither of them had any time off school the whole of last term or this term', and Mrs F said of her daughters, 'Neither of them has had any time off. We've got Clare right through her "O" level mocks without having any time off'. At her third interview Mrs P said that her daughter had been prescribed two courses of antibiotics the previous month for bronchitis. Because she still sounded 'a bit wheezy' when she laughed Mrs P had been keeping an eye on her in case it was necessary for her to go back to the doctor. She went on, 'But as I say at the moment, well, you can hear she's up and down stairs and in and out she seems pretty good on the whole so . . .'. As I will show in a later section, it is this maintenance of normal activity which distinguishes definitions of disorder and definitions of illness.

Defining someone as healthy does not, however, mean that they are free from disorder of any kind. Mrs S, Mrs F, and Mrs G all described disorders their husbands had experienced which did not threaten their conception of them as healthy. At the same time it was also common for them to make statements about their husband such as 'He never complains of anything' or 'He never has anything wrong', when in fact they did on occasions complain and suffer a variety of troubles. This discrepancy I would suggest arises for two reasons, one to do with the nature of the concept of health, the other to do with the nature of the disorders their husbands were seen to experience. Firstly, health is a master status ascribed on the basis of certain features of an individual's biography and is independent of their state at any point in time. 'He never complains' is then a statement about a biography and not a statement about the here and now. Moreover, that biography is not necessarily modified by particular instances where the statement does not apply. This can be contrasted with the definition ill which, at least on some occasions, refers to the here and now. It is possible then to assert that someone is healthy although at that particular point the person is defined as ill.

For example, Mrs S often spoke with concern of her three-year-old daughter, Joanne, who seemed to get repeated throat infections; as she expressed it, 'It's just one cold and bad throat after the other'. When I called to interview Mrs S for the second time Joanne was not well with a sore throat, yet Mrs S was able to maintain that 'Joanne's very healthy apart from the sore throats'. That is, recurrent episodes of this kind do not threaten Mrs S's conception of her daughter's master status since they pertain only to individual here and nows. In Turner's terms, the person conception she holds is relatively stable (Turner 1968). Similarly, when speaking of her father she said, 'Dad was all right apart from his heart, he had angina and hardening of the arteries in his legs'.

Many of the disorders experienced by the respondent's husbands did not challenge their status as healthy since explanations could be found which enabled them to be routinized. As Mrs F went on to say of her husband:

> (F16) (Mrs F) 'He occasionally gets a headache . . . but then I persuaded him to get glasses which he doesn't take to work with him . . . but I think this is all it was, you know . . . I think he gets strained with his job when he has a heavy day and it's very complicated and he's seeing lots of people and talking technicalities and he tends to come home with a sort of sick headache then.'
> (Int.) 'I see . . .'
> (Mrs F) 'But that's . . . it can always be put down to that.'

Here, Mrs F is able to offer reasons for her husband's sick headaches which identify them as part of the normal order of things. Since they are caused by his not wearing his glasses and job strain they are to be expected rather than matters relevant to health. Similarly, when Mrs G says of her husband, 'All he ever gets are common colds', she is asserting that the problems he does get are shared by everyone, are to be expected, and need not be taken into account in making judgements about his health.

I would also suggest that the status 'healthy' is more amorphous than the status 'ill'. It is not a status that has implications for action on the part of the individual or those around him. Defining someone as ill, however, does have practical implications since that individual and those with whom he interacts have to formulate and undertake a variety of actions designed to solve the problems it creates. Illness has to be managed whereas health can be taken for granted. Contrary to Dingwall's suggestion based on the work of Sacks, health, normality, and ordinariness do not constitute the same kind of practical problems as illness or deviance. They require to be displayed only when challenged (Dingwall 1976:67–76). This is, perhaps, the reason why accounts of health are usually less complex than accounts of illness and the reason why we know more about what Dingwall has called ethno-illness than we do about ethno-health. There is just more to know. This would affirm the conclusion often drawn from ethnographies of non-industrial societies; that is, a culture is likely to contain a more detailed and complex body of knowledge about those phenomena which present themselves as practical problems than it is about those which do not.

Definitions of disorder and definitions of illness: maintaining normal activity

Implicit in much of the analysis so far is the distinction I have drawn between definitions of disorder and definitions of illness. The former definition is applied when the problematic experience involved does not result in a concerted change in activity. Mrs P, talking about one of the episodes of bronchitis that affected her daughter, said, 'She had this rattly cough, terrible at night you see, really aggravating then. But in herself she was OK, it didn't put her off eating or anything like that'. At the previous interview she described how her son had 'A mild dose of tonsillitis' the week before; 'he had just a shortish course of antibiotics and er . . . he wasn't ill with it'. Mrs P had not known about the tonsillitis until Martin told the doctor about it at one of her daughter's visits. I take it that Mrs P had not been alerted to the problems because it did not lead to any modification of his behaviour.

Some problematic experiences the respondents talked about were not located within the category 'illness' because of the way they had arisen. For example, though Mrs R's daughter had recently been taken to hospital the problem was not defined as an illness:

(R23) (Int.) 'Have your children had any problems since I last saw you?'

(Mrs R) My daughter fell over and hurt her leg . . . and er . . . but that's not an illness, that was an accident and she went to hospital to have the leg dressed.'

Mrs S employed a similar rationale while attempting to define in more general terms what she would include in the category illness. I had just asked her about her own health:

(S27) (Mrs S) 'I don't have any illnesses, mine are the sort of thing I've got now, I'm not ill, I never get ill, the only thing I have are pulled muscles which can happen to anybody. I always call illnesses something that you get, if you know what I mean, not something you do, get me, something that . . . well an illness as far as I'm concerned is erm . . . I don't know, well I wouldn't call a pulled muscle an illness anyway . . . I'd just call it something I've got which I'll get rid of in two or three days.'

At the interview she made a similar statement while talking about her friends some of whom always seemed to have something wrong with them:

(S28) (Mrs S) 'One of them said to me you never seem to be ill or anything like that. I said I'm not actually ill. I can't call having a pulled muscle ill or having nerves ill, you know, it's just something you seem to suffer with.'

For Mrs S, the type and origins of the problems she encountered influence the definitions she applies. Illness is 'something you get, not something you do'. There is, perhaps, more to it than that. At three of the interviews Mrs S talked about her nervous problem and at one we discussed the effect it had on her:

(S29) (Int.) 'Still getting out and about?'
(Mrs S) 'Yes, oh yes, I mean nothing, it's nothing like that you know ever stop you doing anything. I went to the Ideal Home Exhibition on Monday, I went there the whole day sort of thing, you know, nothing stops me from going anywhere. I just carry on as normal. It's not stopping me from doing any work, I still do it.'

The sorts of disorders which Mrs S experienced from time to time were not problems which limited her activity or affected her ability to carry on 'as normal', she was able to go out and do her housework. Because her problems did not constrain her in any way they were not classified as instances of illness; rather, they were merely something she 'suffered'.

Illness-relevant behaviours such as staying at home or going to see a doctor are not only imposed on the sick they are also actions which convey particular benefits. As Mrs R said of her husband after he was admitted to hospital during an acute phase of his depression, 'he was removed from everything, from his responsibilities and even the children playing around in the evening'. Consequently, these actions may be prescribed when someone claims to be feeling ill. When Mrs R's son complained that he was unwell he was told to go to bed and Mrs S was advised by a friend to go and lie down when she complained of feeling sick. Because anyone complaining in this manner is expected and obliged to undertake these prescribed activities a refusal to comply may mean that their claims are challenged. This may take the form of a charge of irrationality; when Mrs F's mother complained of a tremor in one arm Mrs F suggested she go to the doctor ''cos it's silly to keep on complaining or worrying', or it may lead to a denial of the right to complain. At one time, Mrs R's husband frequently complained of stomach ache and indigestion:

(R24) (Int.) 'He's not thought of seeing the doctor about that?'

(Mrs R) 'Well, yes, I have suggested it to him when he's complained for long periods, erm, but he doesn't want it, he says he doesn't want to start having stomach X-rays and all the rest of it so I'm afraid once or twice I've said all right shut up about it, you know.'

Alternatively, it may be assumed that nothing much can be wrong if the individual concerned is not prepared to suffer the inconvenience of appropriate activities.

However, refusals to see the doctor do not threaten the status of a complaint where acceptable explanations are available to account for that refusal. Just prior to my fourth interview with Mrs P her husband had begun to complain that he was depressed. He had been treated for 'a sort of breakdown' some years previously but this time he refused to go to the doctor:

(P16) (Int.) 'How's your husband?'

(Mrs P) 'Depressed.'

(Int.) 'Is he?'

(Mrs P) 'Mm . . . he ought to go to the doctor but he won't got so . . .'

(Int.) 'You can't persuade him to?'

(Mrs P) 'No. I know if I was to phone Dr M and tell him immediately he'd say send him up to me and I'll put him on some drugs again but he won't go.'

(Int.) 'But you think he ought to be seen by Dr M?'

(Mrs P) 'Well, you see, why he won't go back is probably because he thinks Dr M will send him off to the place where he had treatment before you see, he had electric shock treatment.'

(Int.) 'Yeah. He's not very keen on that?'

(Mrs P) 'No.'

Despite the fact that Mr P's depression had no externally observable manifestations and Mrs P knew nothing of it until he told her, his reluctance to see the doctor is not taken to mean that his claim is dubious nor does it lead to attempts to silence his complaints. Rather, Mrs P formulates and accepts an explanation to account for his refusal to seek medical treatment such that his definition of what is going on is not challenged. This is couched in similar terms to that offered to and rejected by Mrs R; that is, a desire to avoid anticipated consequences of professional help.[3] Similarly, Mrs F's mother's consistent refusal to see the doctor for her many complaints was seen to be the product of a general personal tendency, 'She's got this very old fashioned idea of doctor as God and God mustn't be bothered not unless you're really dying you see. She'll do anything rather than go to the doctor', and did not signify that her complaints were illegitimate.

Though a failure to engage in situationally appropriate behaviour may lead to the repudiation of definitions of illness, the respondents did sometimes assert that they or others known to them had been ill although usual activity was maintained. Mrs S managed this discrepancy by invoking her status as a housewife:

> (S30) (Mrs S) 'If I'm ill I don't go to bed or if I feel poorly I don't I just carry on because if you've got children you can't you just, you just work and carry on and I find mostly that it makes me feel a darned sight better. And Mike can't afford time to be off work to look after me if I was poorly anyway, so I think you'll find not just me but most of the housewives among my neighbours just carry on as we are and get on with it.'

Mrs S's status as a housewife imposes obligations that rule out the possibility of her engaging in what otherwise would be situationally appropriate behaviours. Her responsibility for her children means that she must carry on as usual and 'get on with it'. This is not peculiar to her but is a general situation common to others who occupy a similar status, 'you'll find not just me but most of the housewives among my neighbours just carry on as we are'. Role responsibilities are thus given precedence over those behaviours customarily expected of the sick; consequently the definition ill is not subsequently challenged. That this is taken to be an adequate explanation of the failure to display illness-relevant behaviours requires that commonsense knowledge of social statuses and their attendant obligations is used to recognize the sorts of constraints imposed on those who occupy the role of housewife. Mrs S also appeals to features of the organization of her family to reinforce the conclusion that her maintenance of normal activity is imposed on her and not therefore an indicator of an illegitimate claim to the definition ill. As she explains, her husband would not be able to forgo his responsibilities with regard to work to be able to look after her if she was not well. The need for the major participants in the family to fulfil their obligations in order to maintain it as a functioning unit legitimately prevents the expected change in usual activity.

In a subsequent interview Mrs S reaffirmed this rationale while discussing her parents' response to problematic experiences. The need to look after children is offered as an explanation of the difference in reaction on the part of her mother and father. It is also elevated to a general proposition to account for the differences between men and women:

(S31) (Mrs S) 'My mother was always quite a poorly person, she never was very well, you know, and yet she was marvellous, she would get on with whatever she was doing no matter how she could be at death's door nearly, but if my father was ill he was, that was it, he'd just sit down, I mean he'd just have a pain in his little toe and I think nine men out of ten are just the same. This is how I find it because they never have children to look after. If you've got kids you can't afford to be ill.'

Here, responsibility for children is seen to impose a constraint only on women. While women, like her mother, carry on despite the fact that they 'could be at death's door', men are not limited in this way and are able to dispense with normal activity for relatively trivial conditions. Not only does this account rationalize a discrepancy that might obviate any definitions of illness, it also illustrates the moral superiority of women who place obligation before self-interest. As Mrs S says of her mother, 'she was marvellous'.

Biography as context

In the previous sections I have shown how what I have called illness-relevant behaviours are used in the construction of definitions of health and illness. I have attempted to specify some of the interpretive procedures employed and outlined some aspects of commonsense knowledge about health and illness used as an interpretive scheme. Illness-relevant behaviours are not only included in descriptions of episodes of illness but are invoked to demonstrate the legitimacy of the application of this construct. Although the presence or absence of illness-relevant behaviours is frequently adequate for the task of constructing definitions, it is also the case that more complex rationales may be employed. For example, these behaviours may be situated within a biographical context. In this section I will use further data to show how biography as context functions as an interpretive device. Consider the following exchange:

(G20) (Int.) 'Can you remember the last time that you or anyone you know was ill?'
        (Mrs G) 'Yes, my dad.'
        (Int.) 'When was that?'
        (Mrs G) 'About two months ago.'
        (Int.) 'What was wrong with him?'
        (Mrs G) 'He had sciatica.'
        (Int.) 'Tell me about it. What happened?'
        (Mrs G) 'The reason I remember it probably more than anything

is the fact that he's never . . . I can't remember a time before that when he was ill. I can't really ever remember him going to a doctor's before that. Er . . . he had this severe pain in one of his legs and er . . . *had* to go to the doctor's to get something. But obviously, apparently it's something that he can't sort of give you tablets for and it goes away. You know he had time off work . . . it's just something that . . . extraordinary, non-typical of him.'

What is to be noted in this extract is that Mrs G's depiction of her father as ill does not rest on a description of the disorder as such but other matters are introduced to convey the meaning of the event. That is, the symptom, 'a severe pain in one of his legs', the diagnosis, 'sciatica', and the nature of the disorder, 'it's something that he can't sort of give you tablets for and it goes away' are situated within other facts deemed relevant to the categorization of the event. These other facts consist of the behavioural consequences of the disorder and their location in a biographical context.

When asked to elaborate, Mrs G offers reasons why she can remember this particular event. This takes the form of biographical information; she cannot remember her father ever being ill nor can she really remember him ever having to consult a doctor. This medical history provides a context by means of which the disorder under discussion can be interpreted. It not only serves to convey the uniqueness of the event in question, it also allows her father to be identified as a particular type, as someone who is never ill and who never consults a doctor. This typification is reaffirmed when she says that his having time off work is 'extraordinary . . . non-typical'. On the basis of this typing other relevant characteristics can be imputed to him such as typical courses of action and their motivational and intentional antecedents. Consequently, the fact that on this occasion he 'had to go to the doctor's to get something' and 'had time off work' constitutes grounds for seeing this 'severe pain in one of his legs' as particularly significant. Given what is known of her father in terms of a type, grounds also exist for establishing the nature of the connection between these events. That is, seeing the doctor and taking time off work are the inevitable consequences of an organic disorder. Consequently, the claim to be in pain and the subsequent course of action cannot be seen to be specifically motivated. Although pain, because it is not subject to direct observation, may figure in many illegitimate claims, there is nothing in this description that can be taken as evidence of malingering or exaggeration. This is ruled out by the commonsense association between a type and the kind of motives known to inform their actions. Given that the facts of the matter are presented in this way it would be difficult to question Mrs G's definition of her father as ill.

The reasoning involved in the imputation of illness made here is more complex than those previously analysed. Both make reference to a commonsense construct of how ill people behave and identify these behaviours as the product of a biological disorder or the experiences to which it gives rise. In this instance, however, they are contrasted with the subject's biography *vis-à-vis* doctors and work and the typification thus invoked reinforces the interpretation of these behaviours as signifying illness by providing for the ascription of appropriate motives.[4]

These features can also be discerned in the following exchange taken from another interview with the respondent quoted above. The two interviews were carried out exactly one year apart and in both extracts the respondent's father is the subject of the discussion:

(G21) (Int.) 'What's your father's health like?'
     (Mrs G) 'I think it's very good. I sort of can't remember him being seriously ill. Actually, the first time I've known him have time off work was about a couple of months ago when he had flu, and he must have been bad because he had a good week and half off, he saw the doctor and got a sick note and everything, but that's the only time I can ever remember him, you know, in years, sort of thing.'

The biographical information presented here is somewhat similar to that in the previous example. The respondent cannot remember her father being seriously ill, and the only time that she can remember him having time off work is the occasion she goes on to describe. The sciatica episode is not invoked here, it is either forgotten or has not significantly modified her conception of his biography. Whatever, given this conception of her father's normal pattern of activity having a 'good week and a half off work' and 'seeing the doctor and obtaining a sick note' are taken as indicators that he 'must have been bad'. The connection between these events as indicators, the biography as an interpretive scheme, and the underlying pattern to which the indicators are thus taken to refer are not made explicit in the respondent's talk. The expectation is that reference will be made to a stock of knowledge at hand to fill in and make the necessary connections. This seems to require a more complex interpretive procedure than that suggested by Garfinkel (1967) in his discussion of the documentary method. For taking time off work and going to see a doctor are not unambiguous as indicators. They may also be interpreted as motivated acts, i.e., indicative of malingering. Hence the necessity to warrant the connection being made by the invocation of biography. However, in order to function as an adequate interpretive scheme the biographical facts offered need to be embellished. They are themselves documents of an underlying pattern consisting of types of persons, their actions, and the motives that generate them. Thus, for the purpose at hand persons can be divided into two types, malingerers and non-malingerers. Inferences about observable actions such as staying away from work and seeking medical advice can be made on the basis of the motives known to inform the behaviour of these types. This involves a commonsense theory of the basis of action and constitutes work necessary for the imputation of illness.

The respondents I interviewed not only used aspects of biographies in constructing and legitimating definitions of illness, they also clearly expected anyone they assumed to be in possession of biographical information to use it to arrive at the same interpretations. The following extract illustrates this expectation. It is taken from a part of an interview in which Mrs F describes changes in the organization of her doctor's practice of which she did not approve. Those changes consist of the introduction of receptionists and an appointment system. The account is offered as an illustration of the way in which her doctor's practice had become more impersonal:

> (F17) (Mrs F) 'This is a barrier and . . . I feel quite annoyed about it really, because I don't know if I mentioned it before, my husband is really fit, luckily, for years and years, well I think all our married life, I think all he ever went to Dr M for was an examination prior to taking out an insurance policy, and he had very bad flu, it's the first time he's been ill since we've been married, and I couldn't get the doctor to come and see him. OK, so everybody has flu, but he had a high temperature for about three days and all I got was the receptionist fending me off. Oh well, you can call in for a prescription, you know, sort of describe his symptoms and I'll give you a prescription and this I was so annoyed about because I felt that if Dr M and his old receptionist had been there the only two there they would have thought Mr F never ever comes near us, he must really not be well, or even if he's, it's only flu and he'll get better, we owe him a visit.'
>
> (Int.) 'Yes . . .'
>
> (Mrs F) '. . . you know, for all these years that he hasn't bothered us, and that has made me very resentful.'

Many of the procedures analysed above are readily discernable in this account. While the respondent believes that the request for a visit from the doctor was justifiable on clinical grounds, 'so everybody has flu, but he had a high temperature for three days', she anticipates that the doctor and his old receptionist, knowing her husband's biography as she describes it, would have been competent to recognize that a request for a visit means that 'he must really not be well'. Or even if a visit was not warranted on clinical grounds, knowing the kinds of demands he had made on them in the past the doctor would have recognized an obligation to comply with his demands. The new receptionist who was not in possession of this knowledge is clearly not considered competent to judge whether or not a visit by the doctor is required, though ultimately it is her decision. In this instance a visit by the doctor was not forthcoming and resulted in annoyance and resentment on the part of the respondent. As she emphasized later in the interview:

'As I say, in that particular incident with my husband, Dr M, knowing that he'd never been to him in all those years would have come to see him. He would have known that this man must be ill if he's asking for a doctor because he's never been to us, never bothered us. Under the new set-up with three bustling receptionists with their overalls on and three doctors in the practice, who knows the individual any more?'

Here, knowing the individual is taken to be the basis of good medical practice. Only by knowing the individual can the doctor make proper inferences about his patient's state of health and thereby make competent decisions as to how to act. The growth in the size of her doctor's practice and the increasing complexity of its organization are identified by Mrs F as constraints upon the extent to which the individual can be known. The new set-up either prevents the patient gaining direct access to those in the know, 'all I got was the receptionist', or prevents the personnel involved in the practice from getting to know their patients, 'who knows the individual any more?'

It is possible to discern within the interviews that I conducted two distinct types of biography invoked by the respondents in depictions of matters of health and illness. One I have illustrated via the extracts above which is used to typify individuals in terms of routine patterns of illness-relevant behaviour. The other I will refer to as a diagnostic biography since it makes reference to diagnoses and not to actions conventionally associated with illness. These diagnostic biographies are used in much the same way, as interpretive contexts for assigning a health status or otherwise ordering observed events. Though the data I have collected is insufficient to be definitive, analysis of some of the extracts in which diagnostic biographies occur does point to a status intermediate to health and illness:

(R25) (In an interview I conducted with Mr and Mrs R they gave me the following information about Mr R's father.)

(Mr R) 'You'll shortly meet my ailing dad by the way who's come to do wallpapering with me. You know, he has this . . . he's been terribly ill for twenty-five years or . . . well, more in fact . . .'

(Mrs R) 'As long as I've known him.'

(Mr R) '. . . since about 1936 he's been very ill and it isn't hypochondria, I mean he has genuine illnesses. He has if I have the right name for it diverticulitis and he has erm . . . hiatic hernia he has erm . . .'

(Mrs R) 'He's had a heart attack.'

(Mr R) 'He's had a heart attack and he has . . .'

(Mrs R) 'He has colitis . . .'

(Mr R) 'Yes, nasty colitis.'

(Mrs R) 'Very nasty that.'

(Mr R) 'And so about every other night my mother tells me he, he, you know, he practically went last night sort of thing. But he's another creaking gate who's been going along for years and today he's feeling well and today he's been down here helping with the wallpapering.'

(N7)   (Mrs N) 'Oh, my mother's not a very healthy person.'

(Int.) 'Why would you say that?'

(Mrs N) 'Well, she has so many things wrong with her.'

(Int.) 'Like what?'

(Mrs N) 'Well, she has very bad osteoarthritis and that is really terrible. She's having treatment about three times a week for that and she's had many operations . . . it's a very long story.'

(Int.) 'Does she find that very restricting?'

(Mrs N) 'Well, she's in constant pain. She is a source of worry because of her operations and troubles that she has.'

(Int.) 'So you don't think her health is particularly good?'

(Mrs N) 'I should say physically she's OK . . . no, I don't know how you would put it with her, she's one of these old cracked lags that keeps going. She doesn't look a sick woman when you look at her but er . . . terrible trouble.'

(Int.) 'I see, it's not a disease that er . . . I mean you wouldn't immediately strike you as being, you know, she wouldn't immediately strike you as being ill if you sort of saw her until you actually knew that there was something wrong with her.'

(Mrs N) 'Well, no but . . . well she's had been, was in hospital for nearly a year with another complaint and we get hospitals and umpteen operations . . . we have this worry.'

(R26)   (Int.) 'What's your mother's health like?'

(Mrs R) 'Not very good.'

(Int.) 'Not very good? Why do you say that?'

(Mrs R) 'She has various complaints including very high blood pressure and she's on medication all the time trying to keep it within reasonable limits . . . and she tires very easily, she had a heart attack about eleven years ago, a slight one, and she has generally been quite er . . . she's supposed to be careful, put it that way, I don't think she is particularly, she has to take it a bit easy . . . she has various other minor complaints; well not so minor . . . things like Reynaud's disease and

. . . well I can't think of any of the others at the moment but she's not a very healthy person.'

(Int.) 'Mm . . . so do you find she's quite restricted in what she can do?'

(Mrs R) 'Well . . . [laughs] this is our family joke, we, we . . . not really, she does an awful lot really . . . well, the . . . in fact she leads a perfectly normal life. No she doesn't restrict herself.'

These three cases share the following features: the respondents provide a catalogue of the disorders from which the subjects under discussion suffer; these diagnostic biographies are taken to be relevant in assigning the subjects to a health status; the potential conflict between the diseases listed and their consequences is managed by the use of a category I will call 'not healthy' which defines a master status.

Mr and Mrs R offer a number of diagnoses to support their contention that Mr R's father 'has been terribly ill for twenty-five years . . . or more'. His status is thus defined by his biography and not by his current situation; 'today he's feeling well and today he's been down here helping me with the wallpapering' is to be seen within its biographical context and is not the criterion according to which he is to be judged. Here, the present takes its meaning from the past and does not alter the meaning of the past. 'Today he's feeling well' is to be read as a temporary state within an overall master status and is not an indicator independent of that status. Similarly, Mrs N provides a diagnostic biography for her mother on the basis of which one is expected to make relevant interpretations. The fact that 'she doesn't look a sick woman when you look at her' is not to be employed as an indicator but is to be situated within her history of 'very bad osteoarthritis' and her 'umpteen operations'. Mrs R also assesses her mother according to her biography of 'various complaints' rather than according to the fact that 'she leads a perfectly normal life'. In this way the respondents not only provide interpretations but provide for them by supplying the interpretive scheme to be employed and denying the relevance of indicators which could lead to alternative conclusions.

However, it is not clear from these accounts whether the individuals described should be defined as healthy or ill for certain discrepancies occur which violate our commonsense conception of illness. Note that in two of the cases I assumed following the presentation of the respective biographies that the individuals concerned would be restricted in some way. Yet Mr R is able to assert that his father has been terribly ill for twenty-five years or more although 'today he is well'. Mrs N claims that her mother has 'terrible' osteoarthritis but does not 'look a sick woman', and Mrs R's mother has a variety of 'not so minor complaints' yet leads a perfectly normal life. The contradictions that these statements embody are managed by assigning the subjects a special status. Mr R's father is a 'creaking gate who's been going along for years' and Mrs N's mother is one of these 'old cracked lags that keeps going'. Mrs R manages the discrepancy in her mother's situation by characterizing it as 'our family joke' and defining her as 'not a very healthy person'. Consequently, the behaviours seen as appropriate to illness do not necessarily apply; 'she has to take it a bit easy' and 'she's supposed to be a bit careful' can be seen as the behavioural prescription for this intermediate category, 'not healthy'.[5]

Motives, morality, and the attribution of responsibility

In the preceding analysis I have touched upon the relevance of moral and motivational concerns to the construction of definitions of illness. In this section I want to consider in more detail issues of morality, motivation, and responsibility.

In the following extract, these issues are central to the way in which Mrs G defines her grandmother's problems. What is to be noted is how Mrs G constructs a denial that her grandmother is ill while admitting that she does suffer from a number of disorders:

(G22)　(Int.) 'What about your grandmother?'

(Mrs G) 'You could write a book on her.'

(Int.) 'Why, does she have a lot of problems?'

(Mrs G) 'Well she's . . . she was unusually healthy till about twelve years ago when my grandfather died and she decided that she was . . . that this was the end, and so sort of arthritis, you know, and she suffers from blood pressure as well, she has tablets . . . she has more tablets than . . . I don't know what they're called but she takes a lot of tablets a day.'

(Int.) 'Would you describe her as being ill?'

(Mrs G) 'No.'

(Int.) 'Why not?'

(Mrs G) 'Well, I think that it's more through her own cause that she's ill rather than . . . fair enough, perhaps she's . . . she had cataracts on both eyes which she had operated on . . .'

(Int.) 'What do you mean her own cause?'

(Mrs G) 'Well, more than if she'd . . . well that she gave up . . . rather than anything else.'

(Int.) 'Do you mean that there's nothing really wrong with her or . . .'

(Mrs G) 'Well, the fact that her joints have gone stiff because she's not used them very much . . .'

(Int.) 'You think that she has got one or two things wrong with her but that she's brought them on by her own actions?'

(Mrs G) 'Yes, I do.'

(Int.) 'Is she at all limited by any of her problems?'

(Mrs G) 'Not really, no . . . she's . . .'

(Int.) 'Can she get out and about?'

(Mrs G) 'Yes . . . I mean she wouldn't walk very far now because, erm, it's so long since she did walk a great distance, but she can do. You know she can walk, I mean she can walk. But she's not particularly bothered about it she . . . you know even on a nice day she doesn't really want to walk into the garden or anything.'

Though the respondent provides a catalogue of her grandmother's problems, 'sort of arthritis . . . and she suffers from blood pressure . . . she takes a lot of tablets a day . . . she had cataracts on both eyes which she had operated on', these are not adequate in themselves for the purpose of ascribing or denying illness. Typically, other matters are introduced to facilitate the construction of definitions. In this case the respondent is able to deny that her grandmother is ill by constructing an explanation of her grandmother's problems which renders that definition inapplicable. This is achieved by invoking moral responsibility and seeing these problems as the product of her own actions: 'it's more through her own cause that she's ill'. In refusing to characterize her grandmother as ill Mrs G does not claim that 'there is nothing really wrong with her' (to use the interviewer's formulation) but that problems such as 'stiff joints' stem from the fact that she has not used them very much. This failure to use her joints does not have its origins in a pathological condition preventing her from walking, 'I mean she can walk', rather, it is lack of motivation on her part: 'Even on a nice day, she doesn't really want to walk into the garden'.

This attribution of moral responsibility is based upon what the respondent considers to be inadequate motivation. The problems under discussion are depicted as states of affairs that might have been, and might still be, otherwise. That her grandmother's limitations, inadequate motivation, and moral responsibility are connected is made explicit by the respondent when she presents further biographical information. That is, her grandmother was 'an unusually healthy person' until her husband died and she 'decided that this was the end' and 'gave up'. The lack of normal motivation imputed later in the interview is both product and indicator of her having given up. This response to her husband's death, which was neither inevitable nor outside her control, is identified as the point at which her health problems began. The expectation that the bereaved will eventually return to normal activity can be used to construe the grandmother's response as unreasonable, as indicative of a moral defect and an unjustifiable state of affairs.

As Parsons (1951) has suggested in his analysis of the sick role, persons who are ill are not usually held responsible for their condition, they cannot be blamed for it. Even where they may be held responsible for having exposed themselves to a particular condition, having contracted it they cannot be expected to get rid of it by willpower. This feature of commonsense reasoning about illness is integral to Mrs G's denial that her grandmother is ill. The problem selected to warrant the denial of illness, stiffness of the joints, is not only seen to be something for which she is responsible but the nature of her responsibility, lack of motivation on her part to lead a 'normal' life, means that her condition is resolvable by her own actions. The commonsense association between illness and responsibility is here used as a resource to legitimate the respondent's refusal to grant her grandmother the status 'ill'.

The respondent is not only able to construe her grandmother's disorders as the direct result of motivated actions, she is also able to interpret her claim to be ill as a motivated act. In the subsequent exchange, the respondent provides further grounds for rejecting this claim:

> (G23) (Int.) 'Do you think she thinks of herself as being ill?'
> (Mrs G) 'Oh yes, definitely. Yes.'
> (Int.) 'Why?'
> (Mrs G) 'Well she, you know, I mean . . . she's eighty-six and sort of a lot more fit than most people of that age. And yet you ask her if she's well and oh no, you know, she's never well. And yet she's not, you know, she's not . . . well she doesn't appear to be ill.'
> (Int.) 'So what do you think underlies her saying that she's not well?'
> (Mrs G) 'Well, probably she wants sympathy or something.'
> (Int.) 'Do you give it?'
> (Mrs G) 'No' [laughs].

A claim to illness, like any other illness-relevant behaviour, is not unambiguous as an indicator. It may be taken to signify genuine illness or it may, as in this instance, be seen to be motivated by anticipated gains. In determining which of these alternatives the claim signifies, evidence must be sought to lend support to one or other interpretation. Here, two such items of evidence are offered. Firstly, the claim to illness is to be seen in terms of the grandmother's age and her situation with regard to her contemporaries. As the respondent says, 'she's a lot more fit than most people of her age'. This presupposes a conception of what I have referred to as normal disorders. That is, certain categories of persons are expected to experience certain types of disorder as part of the normal course of events. These disorders are characteristic of types of persons or life stages and not indicators of illness. The respondent's grandmother is presented as displaying less disorder than might normally be expected at her life stage yet still considers herself to be unwell. The expectation is that she should assess her own well-being in terms of that of her contemporaries, and this she manifestly refuses to do: 'and yet you ask her if she's well and oh no, she's never well'. Second, the respondent is able to render the claim to illness suspect by noting a discrepancy between that claim and observation. As Mrs G puts it, she does not 'appear to be ill'.[6]

These procedures allow the claim to illness to be seen to be specifically motivated. At the same time the respondent finds no difficulty in supplying a relevant motive. Here she trades on commonsense knowledge of the way in which someone who is ill can legitimately expect other persons to act towards them. If someone who is ill can expect sympathy and support then any illegitimate claim to illness can be seen to be the result of a desire for sympathy and support. In finding this as the motive for her grandmother's claim Mrs G not only construes that claim as illegitimate but absolves herself from any responsibility. Her refusal to give sympathy can thus be seen to be warranted.[7]

In offering the above account I would suggest that Mrs G is constructing a moral condemnation. In his analysis of the commonsense ascription of deviance McHugh (1970) describes two rules upon which moral condemnations of this kind depend. Any behaviour may be morally reprehensible according to the view that potential ascribers of deviance take of the conventionality and theoreticity of that behaviour. Conventionality is ascribed to behaviour that an observer considers might have taken place in some other fashion, that is, it is not behaviour that is inevitable. An observer evaluates the conventionality of behaviour to determine whether it is unnecessary under the circumstances, or whether there are reasons that can be found to support it. Those reasons typically take the form of appeals to circumstance. Theoreticity relates to the extent to which an actor is considered to be aware of what he is doing. A theoretic actor is assumed to know what conduct is relevant in any situation and to intend his action in the light of this knowledge. Consequently, an actor may attempt to defeat a charge of deviance by showing good reasons for why he behaved in a certain way, by denying that he knew the rules governing a particular situation or by denying that the act in question was intentional.

Dingwall (1976) uses the conventionality rule to claim that illness falls under the general category deviance; that is, it constitutes a breach of public morality. As he puts it, 'illness is not in accord with what might reasonably be expected so that the ill person is someone who might have behaved otherwise but has failed to do so'. The previous analysis of illness-relevant behaviours would indicate that this is not the case. Illness-relevant behaviours, although considered to be departures from normal activity, are explained as the inevitable consequences of a biological or experiential state. Illness-relevant behaviours are not conventional behaviours since adequate reasons can be found to account for them. Only where these behaviours are motivated can a charge of deviance be made. In McHugh's terms, Mrs G is able to see her grandmother's limitations as a state of affairs that might have been otherwise and for which no adequate grounds can be found. Since they are self-imposed, the result of defective motivation on her part, they are also intentional. Her claim to be ill can be similarly judged, as behaviour that is not inevitable and an intentional breach of the rules.

During the interviews I conducted with Mrs F we talked extensively about her mother and her mother's problems. Following an operation for a cataract six years previously she had become increasingly dependent and would no longer leave the house on her own. Mrs F, however, was able to interpret this dependence as having origins other than the physical limitations imposed as a result of the operation. Here issues of motivation and responsibility are not so clear-cut due to the explanatory device that Mrs F employs to account for her mother's dependence:

(F18)   (Int.) 'Yes. Anything else with your mother, I mean she seems to be the one we talk about a lot isn't she?'

(Mrs F) 'Well, we're still humming and haaing about whether she should have the other cataract done, she's had one done about six years ago, I think I told you. She had a very bad time because she had this infection and she was in there six weeks instead of a few days and she's never really honestly pulled herself together since. I mean I know now she's eighty-five but then she was what eighty-one and active but from that operation she has not been outside the door ever on her own.'

(Int.) 'No?'

(Mrs F) 'No she just, 'cos she can only see with one eye now because she hasn't had them both done.'

(Int.) 'So although the cataract operation's improved one eye . . .'

(Mrs F) 'Yes, she can never see with both eyes, you see.'

(Int.) 'Yes. It's not really improved her situation much.'

(Mrs F) 'No, because as I say, she won't go out on her own any more . . . if only she . . . I think it's just a personality thing with her really, she's that type of person, she's sort of introvert and withdrawn and it's never . . . she never encourages you to do anything, it's always oh, I wouldn't if I were you. You know, she'd much rather I stayed at home and never went anywhere and never went to a show or anything, you know, if I say to her I'm going to . . . say if I audition for a part and I don't get it and I say "Oh mum, I didn't get the part", she says, "Oh good, now you won't have to go to rehearsals", you know, it's not oh, what a shame.'

(Int.) 'Yes.'

(Mrs F) 'You know it's, it's erm . . . so she's that sort of person so . . .'

(Int.) 'Cautious . . . ?'

(Mrs F) 'Yes. So this has been enough this operation to stop her as I say even ever . . . she could . . . if only as I say . . . I know another woman who is a conductor actually and she's had both eyes, she had one eye done, carried on working, and then she had the other one done, because she can't drive unless she's got, unless she can see with both eyes and she wants to drive because she wants to go round all these orchestras, amateur orchestras that she conducts and she's seventy something but this is a totally different personality you see. She's got something to get up and go for . . .'

(Int.) 'Yes.'

(Mrs F) 'So she gets up and goes, two cataracts, you know. As I say there's my dear old mum she wouldn't even walk round the block to the pillar box, you know, which is on the same side of the road and you can't get lost round a block can you?'

(Int.) 'Not really. I mean you think in fact that she's physically capable of . . .'

(Mrs F) 'Well, she was when she first had it done you see but she's never pulled herself together, I can only see with one eye therefore I am housebound, full stop, you see. I mean I . . . the neigh-bour gets a lot of her shopping and I take her once every two or three weeks to get her pension and a bit of shopping, erm, . . . she comes to me one week-end, she goes to my brother one week-end but she never ever goes anywhere on her own, you know, she's very very, you know, totally dependent now on us. Except that she's still in her own home and managing to do her own bit of cooking and housework and so on.'

In this account age, 'I mean I know she is eighty-five but then she was what eighty-one and active', and physical incapacity are dismissed as explanations of the fact that Mrs F's mother has never been outside the door on her own since her operation. Rather it stems from the 'bad time' she had in hospital since which 'she's never really pulled herself together'. While this implies a defect of some sort the role of motivation and responsibility is ambiguous since Mrs F sees it as a consequence of her mother's personality, as a characteristic of a type of person. It is her personality that prevents her from undertaking those actions of which she is assumed to be physically capable: 'she wouldn't even walk round the block to the pillar box which is on the same side of the road . . . and you can't get lost round a block, can you?'

Mrs F sees her mother as withdrawn and introverted and presents examples to demonstrate the consequences of these character traits. She also contrasts her mother's situation with that of another individual whose case history is essentially similar but who carried on working despite two operations for cataracts, 'but this is a totally different personality you see'. Instead of defining herself as disabled, 'I can only see with one eye therefore I am housebound', this other 'gets up and goes' despite two cataract operations. In this latter case the role of motivation is clear. The conductor, unlike Mrs F's mother, has had both eyes operated on because she wants to do things which require sight in both eyes. Her interests provide the motivation and the necessity for adequate sight. Mrs F's mother, however, has been 'humming and haaing' for the last six years about a second operation that would improve her situation. As Mrs F puts it, she has 'nothing to get up and go for' and is content to slip into a dependent role.

Although Mrs F presents her mother's dependence as a consequence of lack of interest in life and an attendant lack of motivation to make the most of her capabilities, responsibility is not imputed in the same way as in the previous example since this sequence is explained as the product of an internal constraint. Personality is not something over which an individual has control, it is something that must be accepted however irritating the consequences. This account then does not carry the same moral condemnation as G22 since her self-definition and subsequent actions are not intentional but consequential. They may stem from a lack of motivation but they are not motivated by potential gains.

Later on in the interview Mrs F outlined her commonsense theory that posits a relationship between interests, motives, and illness. At most of her interviews she had referred to the fact that she herself, her husband, and her children were 'very healthy'. In the following exchange she offers a theory which accounts for her family's good health:

(F19)   (Mrs F) 'Do you think it equates to leading an interesting life? I mean can you draw any conclusions or did I ask you this last time 'cos I've got a theory about this. If you've got things to get up and do you will fight off illness it is . . .'

(Int.) 'Mm.'

(Mrs F) 'doesn't, you know, assume the major proportions that it does to someone who never goes anywhere and never does anything but sits and knits and watches television.'

(Int.) 'So you think one of the reasons why, why you . . .'

(Mrs F) 'I think we're all healthy because we're all happy and busy . . . I don't think we've got time to be ill.'

(Int.) 'Do you know anyone in fact who, who maybe does less, you know, is less active than your family, you know, who, who does seem to be like this . . .'

(Mrs F) 'Well, not specifically but you get the feeling that people who haven't got very much to do will talk about themselves and their ailments.'

(Int.) 'Yes.'

(Mrs F) 'You know it would never occur to me to if anyone phones up and says how are you, I say oh fine, I mean I could be behind me dark glasses (with my allergy) but I forget to mention it.'

(Int.) 'Yes . . . yes.'

(Mrs F) 'Because I want to forget it and I've got other things more important to do.'

(Int.) 'Yes.'

(Mrs F) 'I'm too busy to be really ill and if I was ill and there was a show to . . . I mean you know it's like it's like actors, I mean how many actors actually drop dead on stage, they never do. I mean they might occasionally drop dead in the wings, erm, you know, is there a doctor in the house thing, but you know they can't afford to be ill because they're too busy and they're too involved in, in what they're doing, it's too important. Unless they're really struck down with some dreadful virus you know.'

(Int.) 'So you think, I mean a lot of people who aren't busy have a tendency to dwell on . . .'

(Mrs F) 'I always feel this at the back of my mind although I can't quote you any specific people I've always had this feeling that we all keep well because we want to be well because we've got things to be well for and if you're unhappy or you're bored or lonely or you know you've got nothing to get up and got out and do, if you have a cold it's the flu, you know if you have a headache it's a migraine, erm, you know everything is that bit worse because you've got no interest to take it off . . .'

The theory presented here consists of a linked sequence of events encapsulated in her statement 'we all keep well because we want to be well, because we've got things to be well for'. Thus, leading a happy, busy and interesting life means that there is a motivation to be well, 'we've got things to be well for' and 'if you've got things to get up and do you will fight off illness'. That motivation has its origins in a style of life which is busy and interesting and fundamentally incompatible with illness. Pursuing these interests is more important than occupying the status 'ill'. Moreover, it means 'we've got no time to be ill' and 'I'm too busy to be really ill'.

Because of life interests and the motivation to maintain them, disorders are not organized as illness by Mrs F and her family in contrast to 'people who haven't got very much to do' who 'talk about their ailments' and allow them to 'assume . . . major proportions'. In the absence of the kind of life she and the members of her family lead, 'everything is a bit worse because you've got no interest to take it off'. Consequently, a cold becomes flu and a headache becomes a migraine. Mrs F sees health and illness as responses to disorders of various kinds, with motivation playing an important part in determining how a person will respond. To a certain extent, then, illness as a response to problematic experiences may be seen to lie within a person's control except in extreme cases such as the instance she quotes with regard to actors who 'can't afford to be ill because they're too busy and too involved . . . unless they're really struck down with some dreadful virus, you know'. Hence Mrs F's disappointment over her mother, who could be more active and independent 'if only' she possessed the appropriate motives and interests.

In lay theorizing, illness and motivation are linked in several ways. First, a lack of motivation to lead a normal life can produce the problems that form the basis for the adoption of the status 'ill'; second, a lack of interests and motivation to maintain those interests can lead an individual to organize disorders that have their origins elsewhere as illness; and third, claims to illness may be motivated by anticipated gains. The first and third of these theories are used by Mrs G in constructing definitions of her grandmother's situation, and the second is employed by Mrs F to make sense of her mother's dependence.

The motivated manipulation of definitions of disorder and illness

Where claims to be disordered or ill are denied, explanations of those claims are frequently formulated in terms of motives and anticipated gains. Mrs G's grandmother was seen to define herself as ill because she wanted sympathy. Conversely, as was also illustrated by this case, denials of illness may also be manipulative, attempts on the part of others to avoid responsibility for the sick. The ambiguity to which such claims are subject provides others with these interpretive and manipulative opportunities.

Claims to be disordered or ill may, then, be subject to a variety of interpretations. They may be accorded factual status or they may be seen to have origins that render those claims suspect. Even where conditions exist that could account for the claim, legitimacy is not necessarily conferred. In these next two extracts I present more data to show how various claims come to be seen as manipulative by the location of motives. In the first Mrs N describes how conditions existed which account for her daughter's claim to be in pain and indicates how the link between those conditions and attributing factual status to the claim is mediated by certain inferences. These inferences are used to provide for Mrs N's subsequent actions and those of her daughter:

(N9) (Int.) 'I remember that you told me that you and your husband occasionally get backaches, have you had any . . . ?'

(Mrs N) 'My younger daughter had terrible backache. I had her down at the doctor for that.'

(Int.) 'Could you just tell me a little about what happened with that?'

(Mrs N) 'Well, she was lying around on the floor and her back got locked and she was in terrible pain and couldn't straighten up. We were going to take her to see an osteopath but what happened was I took her down to see Dr M after a week or so because she said it was going up into her neck and he said that she'd sprained a ligament in her back and fortunately it's cleared up and we haven't had any complaints.'

(Int.) 'Did she find that the pain in her back meant she had to have any time off school?'

(Mrs N) 'No . . . but erm, she didn't do any PE but the doctor said she could have done, it just suited her not to.'

(Int.) 'And it was about a week since she had er the before the pain first came before you went to Dr M?'

(Mrs N) 'Oh I let her have it a bit longer than that because I thought she was having me on a bit.'

(Int.) 'Really?'

(Mrs N) 'Mm . . . then when she mentioned her neck I thought I'd better have her seen to.'

(Int.) 'And did Dr M prescribe any treatment for her?'

(Mrs N) 'None whatsoever. He just said if it doesn't get any better come back in a fortnight . . . well, obviously within the fortnight there was nothing left.'

(Int.) 'And she's had no complaints with her back since then?'

(Mrs N) 'Oh well, usually when it suits her it becomes bad again, you know what I mean?'

Although Mrs N does say that her daughter 'locked her back' and was 'in terrible pain and couldn't straighten up', this was not her original interpretation of the event. She did not take her daughter to the doctor for more than a week 'because I thought she was having me on a bit'. That is, the claim to be in pain was taken to be an exaggeration and not a true description. Although no reason is given in this extract for that interpretation, Mrs N did talk later on about how her daughter was 'going through that awkward phase'. While this interpretation is a justification of the delay in seeking treatment for her daughter, it also provides for Mrs N's strategy for handling the situation. She adopted a wait-and-see attitude, 'I let her have it a bit longer', assuming that her daughter would not persist with a claim that was not genuine. It was only when she began to complain that the pain was spreading up into her neck that this interpretation was revised and Mrs N says 'I thought I'd better have her seen to'. Despite the fact that the doctor did diagnose a disorder, a sprained ligament in her back, Mrs N's original depiction is not to be seen as wholly unreasonable. Subsequent events demonstrate that her daughter is the type of person to indulge in manipulative claims of that kind. Though the sprained ligament was nothing serious, it required no treatment and had 'obviously' cleared up within the fortnight the doctor established as the period required before another consultation was necessary, Mrs N's daughter used the legitimation of her complaint for her own ends. For example, she avoided doing PE at school because 'it suited her not to' even though this was not contraindicated by the doctor. She also invoked the definition of herself as injured and in pain on those occasions when it could be used in pursuing her own ends, 'when it suits her, it becomes bad again'. Mrs N does not see her daughter's subsequent behaviour as the unavoidable consequence of an organic disorder, rather she uses the doctor's definition of the situation to show that it was wilfully undertaken for personal benefit. In McHugh's terms, the behaviour is conventional. It is also theoretic, since Mrs N's daughter is clearly assumed to be aware of what she is doing. In seeing these actions as inappropriate, Mrs N provides for a view of them as deviant and morally reprehensible.

In the final extract, Mrs S describes how, in concert with the doctor she was able to arrive at a depiction of a problem with her three-year-old daughter's right foot. Again, the way in which the problem is depicted provides for Mrs S's subsequent action. It is also the reason for her reluctance to talk about the problem since her daughter was present in the room during the interview:

(S32) (Mrs S) 'I did go to the doctor's, I knew there was something. I've been for Joanne, yes. I should think it's quite important. She started walking with her foot turned in, her right foot . . . so I was getting a bit worried about that so I took her up to Dr M and he said there was nothing wrong, it was perfectly normal . . . mustn't talk about it now . . . said it was just to do with Michael . . .'

(Int.) 'Yes.'

(Mrs S) '. . . you know, everybody taking a lot of notice of him when we go out and all the rest of it, so he said just ignore it and it's been fine ever since.'

(Int.) 'You just noticed that did you?'

(Mrs S) 'Er, yes, yes, she was you know very . . . I'm not supposed to talk about it in front of her but . . .'

(Int.) 'That's all right.'

(Mrs S) 'In case it starts again then you know if she thinks you're noticing it.'

(Int.) 'It's gone now?'

(Mrs S) 'Mm, hasn't had it for ages. It's just the right one. You know, it's been awfully bad, looked dreadful, everybody was noticing it and talking about it so we had to . . .'

(Int.) 'So it was more than you noticed it?'

(Mrs S) 'Yes, yes I knew, we never used to talk about it because we had a feeling it might be this and, er, Dr M said it was. He said he's had this problem before so he said that probably this is the reason. 'Cos it's perfectly normal, nothing wrong with it at all.'

When Joanne started walking with her foot turned in Mrs S was able to formulate an explanation which was subsequently confirmed by the doctor. His diagnosis that the foot was 'perfectly normal' legitimates her view that the problem has its origin in a realm other than the biological. The doctor and Mrs S draw on their knowledge of the family situation and commonsense assumptions about typical modes of childhood behaviour to construct their account of the event. An important feature of the family context in which this behaviour occurred is that Joanne's ten-year-old brother, Michael, is severely disabled. Consequently, much of Mrs S's efforts revolved around Michael and what she identified as his special needs. It would also seem that he was the focus of attention for others; as Mrs S puts it, 'everybody taking a lot of notice of him when we go out and all the rest of it'. Seen in this context Joanne's walking behaviour is to be interpreted as attention-seeking, an attempt on her part to present herself as similar to Michael so that she will receive the same in the way of notice. This explanation is not in fact explicit in Mrs S's description. She presents a shorthand version, 'it's just to do with Michael', which she expects will be elaborated by reference to a shared stock of knowledge about her family and children in general. Though attention-seeking is not men- tioned by Mrs S there is no difficulty in seeing this as a reasonable explanation, since aberrant behaviour on the part of small children and those other social incompetents, the mentally subnormal, is frequently so depicted. Without reference to this body of knowledge Mrs S's account would be incomprehensible.

This explanation of Joanne's behaviour suggests its own remedy. That is, Mrs S is to ignore it. Her reluctance to talk to me about it while Joanne was in the room stemmed from her attempt to follow the doctor's advice. Her action, however, presupposes further knowledge about the basis of children's behaviour. She clearly draws on a theory of behaviour reinforcement to make sense of what she has been advised to do. 'I'm not supposed to talk about it in front of her . . . in case it starts again then you know if she thinks you're noticing it.' This theory is often presented to young mothers who are advised to ignore a baby's crying. Since crying is attention-seeking, once the baby learns that it can successfully command attention by this method it will cry all the more. A professionalized version of this theory has recently been employed in the institutional management of the mentally handicapped.[8]

What is surprising about this account is that it imputes an intent to manipulate the definition of a situation to a three-year-old child. As I have pointed out, children are not usually regarded as so competent. For example, Atkinson (1978) describes the case of a thirteen-year-old boy found hanged at home, in which suicide was not imputed as he was not considered old enough to formulate an intent to kill himself. Attention-seeking as a category of behaviour seems to constitute a special case in which incompetents may be seen to be motivated by a desire to achieve certain ends but cannot be judged to know what they are doing. While the moral status of such behaviour may be problematic, the imputation of such a category constitutes grounds for refusing to treat such behaviour seriously.

Mental illness and motivation: a case study

While issues of motivation and responsibility are relevant in imputing illness to individuals with various physical conditions, they take on even greater significance when the condition under consideration is 'mental'. The reason for this lies in the nature of the manifestations of what is referred to as mental illness. The experiences that come to be defined as the signs and symptoms of mental disorder are behavioural and emotional, entities usually regarded as being within an individual's control. The ascription of mental illness as opposed to malingering may then depend upon whether forces external to the individual can be found to account for any observed behavioural or emotional aberration. The data that I have, though limited in some respects, would suggest that where no such cause can be identified the problem of motivation and responsibility becomes prominent.

During the year in which I conducted the interviews, the husbands of Mrs R and Mrs P were or became depressed. As I have already mentioned in passing, Mr R was eventually treated as a psychiatric in-patient and subsequently attended group therapy sessions, while Mr P, whose depression was a recurrence of a former state, refused to seek professional help.

One important feature of disorders of this sort is that emotional disturbances are seen to occur in the absence of any prior event that might explain them:

> (R27) (Int.) 'And how is he now?'
>
> (Mrs R) 'Erm, he's better than he was, definitely better. He still has his bad times, it's still a bit erratic . . . you know, he can still get very agitated about nothing or depressed about nothing.'

Similarly, Mrs P said of her husband, 'the children couldn't understand why Daddy was so cross, so irritable, and would shout at them for no apparent reason'. That no immediate reason can be identified for these emotional difficulties opens up the possibility of a definition of mental illness. If depression, irritability, or agitation were to follow life events such as loss of job, working too hard, or death of a relative, they may be seen as normal reactions to the problems that people face from time to time. If an explanation cannot be formulated in terms such as these then an answer is required to the question, 'Why does X get depressed for no reason?' The crucial difference in these two cases is that Mrs P was able to find an answer to this question and to identify an underlying cause, while Mrs R was not. Mrs P accounted for her husband's problem as a product of childhood experiences and familial relations. By contrast, Mrs R, despite extensive and elaborate causal theorizing was unable to see the sense of it and locate an underlying order. As she said at various points in the interview, 'I think, why the hell are you depressed, there's nothing to be depressed about', and 'you haven't got any real deep problems so why don't you forget about whatever it is and carry on living'. Although Mrs R did recognize that responses of this kind were unreasonable, her inability to supply a cause, to create order, left her in something of a dilemma. Despite the fact that she accepted that her husband was ill, an ambiguity remained that was not completely resolved by the time I had completed the interviewing. Mrs P, however, evidenced no such ambiguity; she expressed nothing but worry and concern and a desire to get her husband into treatment.

Mrs R's dilemma, and its consequences for the way in which she reacts to her husband's problems, is illustrated in the next extract:

(R28) (Int.) 'And when he gets these bouts of depression do you have to treat him in a special way?'

(Mrs R) 'I don't know, I find this a very difficult one to answer, it's one the psychiatrist asked me and again I . . . he asked me how did I react and I said I couldn't really answer, he, he got a little impatient with me because he felt I should be able to answer and I said I found it difficult to judge myself how I react.'

(Int.) 'Is that because you react spontaneously in a way without necessarily . . .?'

(Mrs R) 'Well, I don't always react the same way you see. He asked me am I tolerant when he's depressed and the answer is yes, sometimes I am and other times no, I'm not, you know sometimes I get fed up and I get irritable with it and I think well why the hell are you depressed, there's nothing to be depressed about which I know is unreasonable because I know it's an illness although I think I have been less so since he's been in hospital and I think I have understood a little bit better what it's like because I've seen so many others there as well you see and eventually although one realizes it's an illness and that the person's not doing it deliberately, you know this intellectually it's sometimes difficult to accept it emotionally and therefore my reactions are not always the same, they do differ.'

While on the one hand Mrs R defines her husband's condition as an illness, that is, as something for which he is not responsible, 'one realizes that it's an illness and the person's not doing it deliberately', on the other hand there are times when she gets 'fed up' and 'irritable' because she can see no reason for her husband's emotional state. Then she finds it difficult to accept that her husband is in some way not responsible for his situation. The ambiguity exists because of the gap between what she knows intellectually and what she can accept emotionally. This split between her intellect and her emotions accounts for her varying reaction to her husband; sometimes she is tolerant and sometimes she is not, sometimes she is able to accept that he is ill and to respond accordingly and sometimes she is not. As I indicated in the analysis of G23, sympathy and tolerance are only appropriate when someone is seen as genuinely ill.

Mrs R enlarged on some of these points in a later interview when I asked her how other people were responding to her husband's depression:

(R29) (Int.) 'How are you finding the response of other people to his problems, I remember you saying when we talked last time about how it's one of those things that people didn't seem to want to mention and didn't seem to want to know about . . .?'

(Mrs R) 'I think a couple of people I happen to speak to or I happen to meet who . . . they know but I know that they know that he's been ill, have spoken a little, well, asked how is he and how's he getting on . . . erm, but I suppose really basically I think, I think that if people haven't had direct experience simply don't understand, you know, I think the general attitude is oh somebody's depressed well he should pull himself together and go to the cinema or go to a party what have you and cheer up and I think this is very prevalent until you really . . . because this was my attitude at the beginning, you know, you haven't got any real deep problems so why don't you forget about whatever it is and carry on living . . . it's difficult to understand, this seems to be outside the person's control . . . that for no reason that anybody else can understand or even that they can understand, they just get very depressed . . . I mean he doesn't know himself why he gets depressed at all, no obvious or logical reason, so you know people don't understand. I don't expect them to because I found it difficult.'

Mrs R sees the general attitude to depression as being similar to her own initial response. That is, emotional problems of this kind are things for which a person can be held responsible and can be expected to effect a remedy by their own efforts: 'somebody's depressed well he should pull himself together . . . and cheer up'. Again, the absence of a cause is invoked by Mrs R to explain this initial reaction of hers. However, those who hold this attitude are not to be condemned since it is something that Mrs R, on the basis of her own experience, expects. If people 'haven't had direct experience' they don't understand, nor can they be expected to understand. Mrs R herself found it difficult to accept that 'this seems to be outside the person's control' and still reacts to her husband on some occasions as though this were not the case. In arguing in this way, Mrs R not only provides an explanation of the general attitude, she also legitimates her own problem in coming to terms with her husband's situation and her occasional denial that he is ill. Obviously anyone, until they have had experience of these matters, would find it difficult to cope.

At the end of this exchange Mrs R encapsulates the cognitive problem with which she and others are faced. Not only is she unable to find or be supplied with a cause to explain her husband's depression, there is no cause to be found, 'that for no reason that anybody else can understand or even that they can understand they just get very depressed'. The contradiction that arises is that making sense of what is going on involves accepting that no sense is to be made of it, even though in most cultures and Western scientized cultures in particular it is anticipated that explanations can ultimately be found for all the phenomena with which members of a society are presented.

One important factor in influencing Mrs R's view of her husband and his problem was the period of time he spent as an in-patient in a psychiatric hospital. She also saw this as bringing about a dramatic improvement in his condition not so far achieved by psychiatric consultations and drugs:

(R30) (Int.) 'What was it about the in-patient treatment do you think that was the most helpful to him? I mean you seem to think that if there was any dramatic improvement it was that that did it.'

(Mrs R) 'It was then . . . it was then . . . I think there were two things I think first of all the fact of just being removed from every-thing . . . erm, as sort of sanctuary that's how my husband put it and also I think the fact that going into hospital he was able to say, "Well yes I am ill", because with this kind of thing I mean he said half the time he wondered was there really something wrong with him or was he just malingering or, erm, dramatizing whatever he felt and the psychiatrist understood this very well when he said to him, "I think it's best if you do go in, then you will acknowledge yourself to be ill". Once having been in this was a very definite statement he is ill.'

Going into hospital was for Mr R, and I have no doubt for Mrs R, a powerful legitimator that this condition was really an illness. It enabled the alternatives, that he was just malingering or dramatizing, to be rejected. These are, as I have indicated, always possibilities 'with this kind of thing' since the issue of responsibility is not unequivocal. Though having hospital treatment constituted 'a very definite statement' that Mr R was ill and allowed Mrs R to begin to see it in those terms, it did not entirely resolve the ambiguity with which she is faced. As she said at the last interview, 'I do get impatient sometimes, I just feel so weary with it, I just feel oh for God's sake when's this going to end even though I know logically he can't help it I still get like that'.

Professional definitions may, then, only partially legitimate self-definitions. What is also of interest in this extract is that going into hospital and needing hospital treatment are assumed to be the ultimate indicators that a person is genuinely ill. The psychiatrist expects that Mr R will use this assumption as a resource in arriving at a definition of his situation.

Although Mrs R attributed the change in her attitude to her husband's problem to 'direct experience' and 'seeing so many others in hospital', she had in fact known of or had contact with other people who had been or were depressed or had had breakdowns. At the end of the interview from which fragment R30 was taken, we discussed several such cases from among her relatives and acquaintances. In one case I was able to raise the issue of willpower:

(R31) (Mrs R) 'One woman I know, I mean she didn't have a breakdown I mean that would be she got as far as seeing the psychiatrist and she saw him I don't know twice, three times, and one day she said she got up and she took all the tablets and put them in the bin and thought right, that's the end of all this rubbish and she was fine.'

(Int.) 'Really?'

(Mrs R) 'Yes, she was living on, I don't know, Librium and Valium and heavens knows what and she thought what is all, why am I taking all this rubbish and she just threw it away.'

(Int.) 'It just took a bit of willpower and er . . .?'

(Mrs R) 'Yes, yes . . . but then she wasn't very bad to begin with although she was depressed and she wasn't herself she didn't get to the stage where my husband, you know, my husband got to where he just couldn't go to work any more and he couldn't face people and he couldn't answer the telephone and this kind of thing, she never got to that stage.'

The woman discussed above is seen to be able to take control of her situation and, in effect, to decide to be well. Mrs R accepts my formulation that all it took was a bit of willpower. However, she denies the relevance of this case for her husband's problem by demonstrating important differences between the two: 'she wasn't very bad to begin with' and 'she didn't get to the stage where my husband got to'. The severity of Mr R's depression means that he cannot be expected to get better by taking a similar course of action. Though on occasions problems of this sort may be brought under a person's own control and resolved by an act of will, this does not define a universal rule applicable to all cases.

Because the attribution of responsibility or motivation means that sympathy and support may be withdrawn and some form of moral condemnation applied, it is in the interests of the individual concerned to refute such attributions when they arise. Mr and Mrs R were able to use Mr R's admission to hospital and the legitimacy it conferred on his illness to challenge the view that he was in any way responsible for his condition. At times Mrs R reacted angrily to suggestions that her husband was responsible for his depression. Commenting on the fact that her parents-in-law wanted their son's admission to hospital to be kept a secret she said:

(R32) (Mrs R) 'I got cross once or twice, I said he hasn't committed any crime, he hasn't done anything shameful, I just don't see why it should be like this.'

As she went on to say, someone admitted to hospital with a heart attack would receive nothing but sympathy and interest from others, 'you know, people running round with flowers'. Here, Mrs R takes her in-laws' desire for secrecy as evidence of the attribution of moral defect and, by implication, moral blame.[9] As with the depiction of the problem that Mrs R sometimes entertained, this ties the condition to the individual concerned and involves judgements regarding moral status and personal competence. Definitions of illness, however, absolve the individual of responsibility for the condition and render such judgements improper.

The commonsense knowledge that it is expected that the interviewer and respondent share and employ in constructing definitions has much in common with Parsons's description of sick role expectations. This does not mean that Parsons's analysis of the sick role has any validity. Rather, it supports the view that the expectations pertaining to the sick role consist of a commonsense construct located within a social systems analysis of illness.[10] Various aspects of this construct were used by the respondents I interviewed as a resource for ascribing illness or otherwise ordering observed events or states of affairs. This would cast doubt on the characterization of the expectations Parsons outlines as a professional typification of how the sick ought to behave (Bloor and Horobin 1975). For these expectations are integral to lay theorizing about illness. This theorizing is used to constitute illness as a social phenomenon and to demonstrate the legitimacy of the definitions applied.

The events or situations to which these definitions are applied are frequently if not always ambiguous, in that their meaning cannot be determined by observing the situation alone. Hence the general procedure of locating these occasions within an interpretive context. Thus judgements about the meaning of events are made by seeing them in concert with a variety of other events, so that underlying patterns can be identified. These judgements and the meanings used to make sense of events are essentially moral constructs: 'All commonsense descriptions and explanations of social action implicitly assume some kind of evaluation and some social response, at least that of approval or disapproval' (Douglas 1971a:153).

Illness is a moral category because it explains and evaluates given states of affairs. It involves ideas about what is desirable and undesirable and about what is appropriate conduct for a given social status. Further, it is a moral category because it involves judgements about responsibility. As Douglas (1971a:167) has said, 'it must be possible for an individual to have chosen to do otherwise or there can be no moral responsibility'. As I have shown, in lay terms a definition of illness implies that potentially socially disruptive behaviour such as staying in bed or requiring social and economic support from others is unavoidable and outside the individual's control. Since it arises out of underlying biological or psychological abnormalities, the conduct associated with the status 'ill' is not to be judged according to imputed motives and goals. Consequently, only where an individual is seen to manipulate a definition of illness in pursuance of personal ends can a charge of deviance be made.

Notes

1. A failure to draw this distinction between disorder and illness allows Stacey (1976) to state that 'only those who feel ill will present for medical attention' when this is obviously not the case. The claim is made on the basis of Field's (1976) definition of illness 'which refers primarily to the person's feelings of pain, discomfort and the like'. Illness is not a subjective state but one of many labels that may be applied to such subjective experiences. Neither these subjective experiences nor a definition of illness is a necessary precursor of the seeking of medical aid.
2. For example, the World Health Organization defines health as a state of complete physical, mental, and social well-being and not just the absence of disease or infirmity.
3. The difference in the way the women respond to their husband's refusal to seek treatment may arise because Mrs P accepted that her husband was depressed; the onset of the condition confirmed what she anticipated could happen on the basis of his biography. Mrs R, however, was unsure of the

legitimacy of her husband's problem since it was seen to be connected to his depression. Mrs R was uncertain whether or not his complaints regarding his emotional state signified that he was genuinely ill.

4. It is interesting to speculate to what extent the nature of the disorder described necessitates this more elaborate rationale. Is it the case that commonsense knowledge about sciatica is not in itself adequate to justify its depiction as illness? Would diagnostic categories such as pneumonia or cancer have required this degree of elaboration? That is, can persons with these types of disorders be assumed to be ill irrespective of their actions and biographies? Answers to these questions cannot be explored to any great extent by means of interview data simply because the degree to which any account is elaborated is partially a product of the interviewer's questioning. However, there is a point in an interview where questions about the respondent's commonsense observations can no longer be made without threatening the interviewer's status as competent member. While it may be justifiable to ask 'Do you consider someone with sciatica to be ill?', a question such as 'Do you consider someone with cancer to be ill?' is likely to violate commonsense assumptions. Consequently, it is tempting to assert that there is a relationship between the nature of the condition described and the extent to which a justification of the imputation of illness can be legitimately demanded. Smith has also suggested that more complex rationales are required to support a definition of mental illness where the behaviours upon which the definition is based could be subject to alternative interpretations. See D. E. Smith (1972).

5. This category would seem to have much in common with what Kassebaum and Baumann (1965) have referred to as the chronic sick role and Gordon (1966) has termed the impaired role.

6. Claims to be ill, like the communicative cues described in the previous chapter, may refer to experiences not observable to others. The absence of this type of verification may be used to cast doubt on those claims.

7. That illness does involve a responsibility on the part of others was often referred to by the respondents. It can be seen in the following data fragment:

> (Int.) 'Now your husband seems to have been unwell . . .'
> (Mrs P) 'Oh yes, he was . . . erm, we went down to Reading on the Sunday and really he shouldn't have gone, he wasn't at all well. In fact, his mother's been so unwell we felt we had to go and see her. That morning he woke up and said, "My chest does feel tight and uncomfortable", and he started to cough and I thought, hello, you know, this is it sort of thing, that tight nasty cough, but as I say we went down anyway.'

Here Mrs P asserts that she and her husband felt obliged to go and see his mother, who had been unwell. 'We felt we *had* to go and see her', even though this was obviously contrary to his own interests, 'he shouldn't have gone, he wasn't at all well'. Mrs R described how a friend, apparently afraid of breaching the conspiracy of silence, had initially been unsure of whether to telephone Mrs R after Mr R had been admitted as a psychiatric in-patient. Mrs R reports her friend as saying, 'I thought, hang it all, if he's ill he's ill and I must phone'.

8. Here, 'appropriate' behaviour is rewarded and reinforced by staff attention while aggressive or disruptive actions are ignored: see Whatmore, Duward, and Kushlik (1974).

9. Despite her not expecting others to understand the problem of mental illness, Mrs R was annoyed and confused by the conspiracy of silence she perceived as surrounding the issue. At one interview she said, 'Why should it be like this?'

10. Parsons does say that the expectations he describes seem 'very nearly obvious on a commonsense level' (1958:177). For a discussion of the construction of Parsons's theory of the sick role see Locker (1979).

6 Illness behaviour: the identification of rational action

In Chapters 4 and 5 I examined some of the interpretive processes involved in the ascription of meanings to various events and situations. In this chapter I attempt to use the same theoretical and methodological approach in the analysis of social action, specifically illness behaviour. This requires prior consideration of two problems: first, the theoretical issue of what sort of sociological understanding of social action is possible; and second, the methodological issue of how that understanding may be developed via the use of interview talk.

There are two distinct ways in which an understanding of social action may be achieved. These can be termed antecedent and non-antecedent approaches. The former, as the name suggests, attempts to identify what are taken to be the antecedents of action. There are two versions of this: a causal version which locates factors prior to and causative of action, typically socio-demographic characteristics, norms, values, attitudes, expectations, and a whole range of other psychological and/or social structural variables; and a non-causal version which sees action grounded in meanings, reasons, and intentions. The former sees man as a passive organism responding to 'external' or 'internal' influences, the latter as an active agent constructing his action towards the world according to the way he defines the situation and his own intentions or purposes in that situation. Both of these schemes are explanatory. Mechanic, while he espouses the latter view in his theoretical writings, resorts to the former in his research practice where he has investigated the influence of a variety of social and social-psychological factors on utilization of medical care. Parsons, however, falls within the causal antecedent approach although system needs, socialization, and occupancy of social roles are identified as the precursors of action rather than a range of sociological or psychological variables. By contrast, the non-antecedent approach does not attempt to explain social action in terms of antecedents but describes the process whereby social action is constituted. Behaviour, and its consequences, take on social and sociological relevance only when subject to interpretation by actors in society. Understanding social action

takes the form of describing the interpretive process via which action
is constituted as a social object.

The symbolic interactionist position employed in Chapter 1 involves a
non-causal antecedent approach and an interpretive non-antecedent
approach. As Blumer suggests,

> '[In interaction] the participants fit their acts together, first by
> identifying the social act in which they are about to engage and,
> second, by interpreting and defining each other's acts in forming the
> joint action. By identifying the joint action or the social act, the
> participant is able to orient himself; he has a key to intepreting the
> acts of others and a guide for directing his action with regard to
> them . . . [The participants] have to ascertain what the others are
> doing and plan to do and make indications to one another of what to
> do.' (Blumer 1966)

Here, the behaviour of others is continually subject to interpretation
and redefinition. The context, itself defined as a particular type of social
act, is used as a scheme for the interpretation of the actions of individual
participants. The meanings imputed to the joint act and to individual
actions are the basis on which actors construct their own actions.
Thus, actors constitute joint acts and the acts of individuals as social
objects through this interpretive process and these meanings become
the antecedents of their own reactions. The symbolic interactionists,
however, have not provided a theory of meaning which describes this
interpretive process, nor have they specified how meanings as
antecedents give rise to action.

Zimmerman and Weider have provided a critique of the view that
meanings are the basis upon which action is built. Meanings are viewed
in much the same way as norms and other imputed attributes, as analysts'
resources for accounting for action. Instead, they suggest that meanings
should become topics for study. This involves the suspension of the
assumption that social conduct is based in meanings and its substitution
by the study of the way in which members go about seeing, describing,
and explaining the world in which they live:

> 'The ethnomethodologist is not concerned with providing causal
> explanations of observably regular, patterned, repetitive actions by
> some kind of analysis of the actor's point of view. He is concerned with
> how members of society go about the task of seeing, describing and
> explaining order.' (Zimmermann and Weider 1971)

The concern here is with the procedures that are used in recognizing,
making sense of, and thereby producing the regularity of, the social and
physical environment. One implication of this position is that there can be
no sociological explanation of social action; ethnomethodology sees man

as a skilled cognitian but not, as recent writers have pointed out, as an actor (Giddens 1976; Smart 1976). What this means is that ethno-methodologists do not theorize about social action, they investigate the practical reasoning presupposed in members' theorizing about social action. Sociological accounts of social action are not taken to be qualitatively different from or superior to commonsense accounts. Sociology merely comprises one set of resources for creating order and regularity in social life; sociological concepts and tacit assumptions are the means by which these regularities are identified and explained.

The interactionist and ethnomethodological positions have impli-cations for the way in which interview talk can be used in the analysis of social action. In the former, respondents' statements are taken to be descriptions of the actor's point of view within which meanings, the precursors of actions, can be located. The latter approach treats re-spondents' statements as phenomena in their own right to be used to investigate the resources employed in the creation and communication of experience. To the extent that both theoretical perspectives accord some degree of significance to the interpretive process, an analysis of the production of meanings contributes to both. As far as the first approach is concerned this is the first step in the analysis of social action, while the second approach would take a description of the interpretive process as all there is to say.

However, the problem posed by interview talk for the non-causal antecedent position is what of substance can be said about social action from accounts that are interpretive reconstructions of past events. As I have emphasized throughout, the interview is one context in which respondents may be called upon to give accounts of their own actions or the actions of others. It is not necessarily the case that the characterization of and rationale for those actions is the same across contexts or time. It is this that makes for difficulties in using respondents' statements as indicators of meanings imputed at given points in time. However, in order to provide an explanation of social action based on meanings, it is necessary to be able to say what meanings were imputed to given objects at given points in time and to show how these gave rise to the action to be explained. This demands the possibility of literal descriptions (Wilson 1971). Or it requires the sociologist to make inferences about what happened and how it happened from respondents' interpretive accounts.[1] The interpretive leaps involved in this process are ac-complished by reference to unexplicited commonsense assumptions about social life. Such is the ethnomethodological critique of conventional methodology. Consequently, accounts of actions cannot be legitimately used to locate meanings considered to be the antecedents of those actions. Just what data would be needed to construct a non-causal antecedent explanation of social action appears to be something of a problem.

As far as the non-antecedent approach is concerned the problem is not methodological but theoretical. While interview talk can be used to describe the processes whereby actions are constituted as social objects, the approach can take us no further. As I have mentioned, it presents a theory of the cognitive organization of social order but denies the possibility of a sociological theory of social action. But as Wilson (1971) points out, action involves much more than the outcome of interpretive processes. In addition, while this approach presents a theory of meaning that theory is incomplete. It may tell us how particular interpretations of events were arrived at, but not why those interpretations rather than others.[2] In some ways the theoretical limitations of this perspective are similar to those entailed by labelling theory. While labelling theory shows how behaviours become constituted as deviance as a result of societal reaction, it cannot explain the origins of the behaviours so constituted.

Irrespective of whether an interactionist or ethnomethodological stance is adopted, an analysis of the cognitive process involved in the constitution of action can be achieved using interview talk as data. It poses less complex theoretical and methodological problems than attempts to get at the genesis of action via the same data. This analysis consists of the explication and clarification of the actor's rationality for his actions and reveals 'the techniques men use to make visible for themselves and others the orderliness of the actions they perform' (Moore 1974:111). For example, Moore (1974) has shown how radical clergymen talk about the Church and the community in ways which identify problems that need to be solved. By indicating how their role qualifies them to assist in the solution of these problems, they provide a rationale for their actions and legitimation for their occupation. Stimson and Webb (1976) have also described how members talk about their encounters with doctors in ways which allow others to see them as sensible and rational actors. In so characterizing themselves and their actions they are able to defeat potential charges that they are odd, deviant, or otherwise abnormal.

Going to see the doctor

During the course of the conversations I had with the respondents they frequently made general statements about how and when they would go to the doctor:

(N10) (Mrs N) 'I don't go to the doctor very often . . . it's only when I have to . . . I don't like to worry him too much these days anyway.'

(S33) (Mrs S) 'I only go when I think it's something I ought to go about. If I know what it is then I don't go because I'd rather not.'

(R33) (Mrs R) 'I don't like to dash up at the slightest thing, you know.'

(P17) (Mrs P) 'I don't go unless I can help it. I'm more prone to take the children, you know, than myself or my husband, sort of thing.'

(F27) (Mrs F) 'I think somehow we look on the doctor more or less as a last resort. I mean for other people I always say go, but if it's for me I think ignore it, it'll go away.'

(G24) (Mrs G) 'If it's something that I can treat myself rather than go up and see the doctor, I'll buy something, you know, cough mixture or something like that.'

These statements are indicative of the fact that the respondents take for granted the rationality of their actions and assume that their use of the doctor is appropriate and responsible. Mrs G and Mrs S, for example, emphasized that they would only consult the doctor if a relatively serious problem arose which they could not deal with themselves.

(G25) (Mrs G) 'If it was something trivial, just minor that made me feel under the weather I'd try and buy something to ease or correct it; if it was something worse then I'd go to the doctor's and see what he could do for me.'

(S34) (Mrs S) 'I don't take the children or ourselves to the doctor unless I think it's something, it's serious enough to go.'

In statements made at other points in the interviews the respondents claimed that they were competent to make decisions about when to see the doctor:

(F22) (Mrs F) 'I was talking to my daughter about this, I was saying, you know, animals you take because you don't know how bad they are, but when it's you, you sort of know whether you're ill or not.'

(G26) (Mrs G) 'Surely most people know, don't they? I suppose with a child you wouldn't take any chances but, I mean, sort of, an adult, surely you know if you ought to see a doctor.'

(R34) (Mrs R) 'I don't think I would be neglectful with the children, erm, with my husband, well, you know, he's an adult, I could only say to him if I were worried about him you ought to go to the doctor and nag him a bit if I think he ought to to . . . I . . . I might be like I am with myself, I might feel, you know, if he doesn't feel he ought to go maybe he needn't . . . with the children I think I would be more careful because I know I've got to make the decision not they and I wouldn't take any undue risks there. I mean, I wouldn't run them round to the doctor every time they sneezed or something, er, but if I thought there were cause for concern then I would.'

In these extracts an adult is depicted as knowing whether he is ill and whether he needs medical attention. Consequently, any visit to the doctor can be seen to be for good and proper reasons. The only exceptions to this rule are with animals and other communicative incompetents such as children. The former you 'take because you don't know how bad they are'. With the latter 'you don't take any chances' or 'undue risks' because, as I have previously suggested, any disorder in a child which is not immediately recognizable as a childhood ailment is a legitimate cause for concern and because children as communicative incompetents cannot always explain fully what is wrong with them. That this may create something of a dilemma was recognized by Mrs R when she said, 'you often don't know what to do for the best'. Refusing to take chances and consulting the doctor in situations where the issue is not clear-cut is one way in which the respondents were able to resolve the issue and demonstrate responsible parenthood.

Not only did the respondents assert that they would not visit the doctor other than for problems which were serious or troubles they could not resolve themselves, they also offered good reasons for this course of action by depicting their doctors as busy individuals who were not to be bothered with trivial matters:

(G27) (Mrs G) 'If I did get a slight ailment I wouldn't go unless I thought it was really worth it . . . probably because you think they're hallowed and you shouldn't waste their time.'

(S35) (Mrs S) 'I always try and sort it out myself before I go to the doctor because I find that, you know, he is pretty busy.'

(S36) (Mrs S) 'If I find they get really bad coughs and colds then I'll go to the doctor but if I can get rid of them by myself then I will. I think they've got enough worries without them having minor coughs and colds.'

Respondents' descriptions of when and why they visited the doctor or took an alternative course of action are justifications. They constitute the materials which an observer can use, and is expected to use, to identify what they did as situationally appropriate and themselves as responsible patients and mothers. This is not to assert that these women indulged in some form of impression management, presenting distorted accounts of events that they know did not happen that way. Rather, it reflects their own belief in themselves as competent actors and decision-makers. It is the breach of this assumption of their own competence which gives rise to annoyance when the appropriateness of their actions is challenged.

Some of the points made above can be illustrated by the analysis of the following extract taken from an interview with Mrs G. In this account she describes a series of events which led her to telephone

·the doctor about her eight-month-old son:

(G28) (Int.) 'Well, tell me about Daniel then. What did you say he'd been to the doctor for?'

(Mrs G) 'Well, he went, erm . . . I rang the doctor on a Saturday lunchtime about one o'clock because he'd been violently sick. He'd had diarrhoea for a couple of days but then with a baby you sort of think, you know, diarrhoea can be caused through anything, can't it, too much fruit or something like that?'

(Int.) 'Why, is it common in babies?'

(Mrs G) 'And then he was really sick, it was while we were out and he was sick all over Habitat's front doorstep, really ill, bad. Came straight back, I rang the doctor but he was at home 'cos surgery finishes up here at twelve o'clock on a Saturday. It was Dr C . . . and I rang him at home and he was sort of ever so funny with me until he said to me, mm . . . you know, he was mad because I hadn't rung before you see but it wasn't obvious that he was ill until then . . .'

(Int.) 'Is that why you say he was funny with you?'

(Mrs G) 'Yes, because it was after surgery hours . . . and he changed the, oh . . . he changed his tune as soon as he said to me, mm "Have I seen this baby before?", so I said yes once at a three month check-up, by this time he was eight months old and that was the first time, you know, that he'd been ill and I'd rung the doctor, and he said "Oh, been remarkably healthy up to now then?" and he changed his tune completely, he realized that I didn't ring every Saturday afternoon.'

(Int.) 'Yes . . .'

(Mrs G) 'But it put me off, it did . . .'

(Int.) 'Off the doctor?'

(Mrs G) 'Yes, it did, yes.'

Mrs G begins by describing how her son had diarrhoea for two days and it was only when he was 'violently sick' that she contacted the doctor. She implies that at the time the diarrhoea was not viewed as being anything out of the ordinary and provides an interpretive scheme by which this conclusion can be reached. Here, she invokes her son's life stage and some typical feature associated with that life stage to construct the meaning of the event. Thus, 'in a baby' diarrhoea can be caused by a range of things and therefore does not always signify illness or call for medical attention. It can point to more than one underlying theme, it could be due to 'too much fruit or something like that'. Given this context and the absence of any evidence to the contrary, the interpretation of the event as routine, as something which happens to babies, is as good as any other. I take 'can't it' not as a question but as an appeal to an observer to see the reasonableness of this judgement. When later called upon to justify her delay in phoning the doctor she makes recourse to the ambiguity of the situation, 'it wasn't obvious that he was ill', at the time. What is more, there were no grounds for defining him that way since the diarrhoea could equally have been a routine state of affairs. It was only when her son was sick that she redefined him as ill and in need of medical care and the diarrhoea as an earlier indicator of that.[3]

In this account Mrs G describes how she interpreted certain events and provides a rationale which allows those interpretations to be seen as reasonable under the circumstances. Though her initial interpretation turned out to be inadequate it cannot be deemed incompetent, given the facts at her disposal. Though the diarrhoea subsequently proved to be an early manifestation of illness, the normal form in which it presented means that she cannot be expected to have known it for what it was at that time. Once some clear indicator was available she had no trouble in imputing an appropriate definition. In this way she is able to present herself as a good mother providing adequate care for a child for whom she is responsible. The account is then a justification of her seeing things in the way that she did and a justification of acting in the way she did. By grounding her actions in the definitions she constructs to make sense of events, Mrs G both explains and legitimates her conduct. Such justifications are necessary lest these actions are subject to the same kind of challenge she reports in her encounter with the doctor. They allow her to maintain an appearance of what Voysey (1975) refers to as adequate parenthood.

I take it that the central feature of this account is the respondent's explanation of her delay called for by the doctor challenging her actions. This is constructed to show that she could not have acted otherwise. The research interview thus provides Mrs G with one opportunity to demonstrate the sense of her actions and reaffirm the competence of her performance as mother and patient. This is accomplished through her ability to show that what she did was reasonable in context and that any attempt to categorize her as incompetent or neglectful is unfounded since it presupposes her to be a type her previous conduct shows she is not. As she was able to convince the doctor, she is not the sort of mother who rings the surgery every Saturday.[4]

This extract also illustrates what seems to be a typical dilemma in the lay management of trivial disorder and the kind of interactional problems it may engender. Where problematic experiences are ambiguous within the context of the knowledge at an individual's disposal decisions as to meaning may be difficult to make. It may not be apparent whether they signify 'normality' or 'illness'. Where such manifestations are seen as indicating that something is wrong, it may not be clear that the condition is sufficiently severe to warrant medical attention. Individuals may then be caught between the alternatives of going to the doctor with a disorder that may be medically insignificant or waiting for future developments with the potential risk that this entails. In both cases charges of incompetence or irresponsibility may result and create conflict in doctor-patient and patient-other interactions. The kind of accounts presented above are integral to the management of these interactions. As I shall describe later, patients often invoke the anticipated reactions of the doctor and the more general decision rules presented above in explaining their failure to seek medical treatment. They also develop strategies for influencing the doctor's reaction when they do present. These represent some of the methods people use for coping with ambiguity and the interactional problems to which it may give rise.

The critical incident

The account given above by Mrs G contains what Cowie has referred to as a critical incident, a physiologic version of Zola's non-physiologic triggers. The cardiac patients Cowie studied identified this critical incident, an increase in the severity of chest pain or the development of other symptoms such as breathlessness or sweating, as the reason for deciding to call the doctor:

'The symptoms before, or at the initial stage of the critical incident were normalised in a variety of ways. They were regarded as indigestion which everybody knows is a non-serious, non-threatening ailment treated by a variety of home remedies, or they were regarded as indicating the occurrence of yet another bout of a previously experienced illness which although it may be serious need not cause alarm as recipes for action in the past had proved successful.' (Cowie 1976:90)

This initial interpretation, as in the example I gave above, constitutes the justification for delay in seeking professional help just as the critical incident is offered as a justification for reinterpreting the situation as serious and consulting the GP. In constructing the justification for the initial delay individuals point to the reasonableness of the interpretation by showing that it fits the available facts. Any moral condemnation or charge of incompetence is then unwarranted since this initial definition is not to be seen as inappropriate.

In previous chapters I have presented cases which can also be used to illustrate this general process, although in these cases the conditions of concern to the respondents were relatively trivial. For example, in data extract N9 (Chapter 5), Mrs N initially interpreted her daughter's claim to have hurt her back as malingering, though this was revised when her daughter began to complain of pain in the neck, and professional help was sought. Similarly, when her daughter was sent home from school with a severe headache, data extract N4 (Chapter 4), Mrs N saw it as a consequence of the glandular fever from which she had recently recovered. However, when her husband came home with the same complaint the problem was redefined and the doctor contacted. Mrs P, in data extract P2 (Chapter 4), initially thought her daughter's complaints of a sore spot on her foot were due to a minor abrasion and it was only when the girl came home limping that she thought she had better have it looked at. In all these cases the original interpretation was such that the problem was routinized and was only seen to be something else following a new incident. In the following example, a critical incident brought about a reinterpretation of a problem that had been present for some months:

(P18) (Mrs P) 'Didn't I tell you I'd slipped a disc? That was at the beginning of this year. Erm, for months the doctor thought I'd had sciatica, I had the pain low down and right through my seat and down this part of the leg and, er, it came and went, I had it for quite a long spell and then it started to clear and it seemed to be better and a couple of mornings I had it again and on this particular morning when I went to get up . . . we'd over-slept a bit and I had this sort of nagging pain low down in my back and down my leg and I thought, oh golly, you know, it's going to be a nuisance today, let's get out of bed quick and I sort of put my hand on the bed and sort of shot myself forward like that which I shouldn't have done and, er, I went into the bathroom and all of a sudden I just screamed with pain, I couldn't move, I've never experienced anything like it in my life. My husband was shaving, it's a wonder he didn't cut his throat. I just felt I've got to scream and I couldn't stop and I just sort of grabbed the towel rail, I sort of turned round against the wall and hung on to this and I just went on screaming and screaming. He said whatever's the matter, oh, I said, my back. I've never had a pain like it in my life before, I really haven't and as I say I know it sounds stupid but I felt I've got to scream to do something, you know. As I say, it's a wonder the lady next door didn't come flying in thinking murder was being done, but the poor kids they came flying into the bathroom, they looked at me shattered, and they sort of helped me back to bed, he sort of gripped me under the elbows and I shuffled out I couldn't walk, I didn't know what had hit me for a minute and of course I let go of him and I literally fell on the bed and he picked my legs up and of course I screamed again, he flattened me out, covered me up and then he phoned the doctor.'

In this extended account Mrs P tells how the pain in her back when she woke one morning was taken to be a reoccurrence of her sciatica for which she had been treated for some months: '*It's* going to be a nuisance today' (my emphasis). Within minutes a critical incident had occurred which in and of itself led to the doctor being called and subsequently brought about a revision of the original diagnosis. As Mrs P says, the doctor initially thought she had sciatica. The character of the new symptoms Mrs P described is sufficient justification for the decision to telephone the doctor. The intensity of the pain, demonstrated by her response, 'I just went on screaming and screaming', and her subsequent inability to walk, was so unlike anything she had experienced before that it could not be routinized by reference to the original interpretation.

As in other accounts, the interpretations applied at any given point in time establish a context in which the respondent's action *vis-à-vis* the doctor is demonstrably rational. However, the connection between the interpretation and subsequent action is not made explicit. An observer must and is expected to refer to a stock of knowledge to make the assumed connection. This involves recognizing the problem described as falling within or outside of that range of situations in which it is appropriate to consult a doctor since he is in a position to offer a solution. In addition, the motives of the respondents in seeking professional help are assumed to be apparent.

Critical incidents were not reported in all the cases in which the respondents sought medical help. Such incidents seem to be the precursor of consultations in those situations in which a feasible alternative explanation is available. In others, in the absence of an explanation which would routinize the problem, the character of the symptoms suggested that something serious was wrong. At one interview Mrs F had just taken her mother to see the doctor 'because of this pain when she swallowed':

(F23) (Mrs F) 'When she swallowed she got this bad pain, so of course she was worried, she immediately thought she'd got this terrible blockage or something dreadful so I took her round to her doctor.'

(Int.) 'So there was none of her usual resistance to seeing the doctor?'

(Mrs F) 'No, no 'cos she was really worried that there was something really wrong.'

At another interview Mrs N's husband had recently been to the doctor to see about a pain in his arm:

(N11) (Mrs N) 'My husband went to see Dr Z because he had a pain in his arm and he thought, God, I'm going to have a heart attack, that's where it starts and I suppose the doctor realized he was the worrying kind and though he couldn't find anything wrong with him he sent him to a specialist for tests who said there's nothing wrong.'

In both of these cases the respondents present the interpretations others apply to their problems as the basis for subsequent actions. The tentative diagnoses applied to the symptoms indicate a potentially serious disorder and constitute the rationale for those individuals behaving in those particular ways. The recognition of this as rational action involves accepting that those diagnoses were reasonable under the circumstances (as it turned out Mrs F's mother had a small oesophageal ulcer which rapidly healed and the doctor could find nothing wrong with Mrs N's husband) and that the individuals concerned were acting prudently in presenting themselves for professional diagnosis. As Mr R says in a similar situation I will describe later, 'I just wanted to make sure'. One of the perceived functions of the doctor is that he alleviates worry by providing proper diagnoses.

In some cases, the character of the symptoms immediately ruled out an explanation which could otherwise have been used to define a problem as routine. Mrs S, as I have described, periodically pulled muscles in her neck, stomach, or back while lifting her handicapped son in and out of his wheelchair. These gave rise to pain and some limitation of movement. Because these were a routine feature of Mrs S's life, something she expected to happen, 'pulled muscles' was available to explain pain or stiffness in any of these locations. At one interview Mrs S described how, contrary to her usual practice, she had consulted the doctor about what turned out to be a pulled muscle in her stomach:

> (S37) (Mrs S) 'I had to go to the doctor with it because it was really nasty and I was a bit frightened it might be something else.'
> (Int.) 'Was that just painful?'
> (Mrs S) 'Oh no, I couldn't stand up. I was frightened it might be appendix or something like that. I was practically bent double with it, it was really very bad.'

In this instance the severity of the symptoms suggested something more serious, such as appendicitis, and the doctor was consulted. Again, the rationale for seeing the doctor lies in the tentative diagnosis originally applied.

The construction of these tentative diagnoses frequently involves the use of knowledge about the typical ways in which certain disorders manifest themselves. When Mrs R was told by her mother that her leg had suddenly become very swollen and painful the previous evening Mrs R advised her to 'go down to the doctor immediately because she has very high blood pressure'. As Mrs R said later, 'I thought it might have been a thrombosis, you know, with high blood pressure this is always a risk'. As it turned out the pain and swelling had gone when her mother saw the doctor and the problem was never definitely diagnosed. However, the sensible character of the action is taken for granted given what the symptoms, in the context of other knowledge, might have indicated. Similarly, Mrs G, who was pregnant at the first interview, thought that a show of blood was the onset of a miscarriage:

(G29) (Mrs G) 'At first I thought it was a miscarriage, you know, the first thing I thought of when I saw the bleeding, it was that . . . then I realised the blood wasn't coming from the vagina.'

This first diagnosis was derived from seeing the symptom, bleeding from the region of the lower abdomen, in the context of pregnancy. Subsequently, when Mrs G decided that the blood was coming from the 'back passage' she thought she had piles and went to the doctor. When I asked her why she had sought professional help Mrs G again invoked the fact of her pregnancy:

(G30) (Mrs G) 'Well, I wouldn't try and treat those . . . I wouldn't try and treat that myself.'
(Int.) 'Why not?'
(Mrs G) 'Well, because I was pregnant. Probably if I hadn't been pregnant I probably would have done, I would have bought something, you know, a suppository or some kind of, er, cream and tried it first before I went. But the fact that I was pregnant made me go and get something which was medically safe to use and effective and also in a leaflet they give out it says that you should let your doctor know if you are susceptible to piles. That was the first time in my life that I'd ever had them.'

By invoking pregnancy and the medically-defined relevance of piles for pregnancy Mrs G is able to show that consulting the doctor about what might ordinarily be a trivial complaint to be handled by self-medication was a reasonable thing to do. In this way she establishes that her consulting the doctor on a specific occasion is consistent with her general statements on the same issue. That is, she only consults for conditions which are not trivial and which she cannot be expected to treat herself.

In constructing initial diagnoses of their symptoms the respondents also made use of a notion of time. That is, both the character and the duration of the symptoms contributed to their definition that something potentially serious was wrong which needed medical attention. When Mrs G had a 'real sort of bad pain in my stomach' the duration of the symptoms ruled out routine diagnoses:

(G31) (Mrs G) 'So after a couple of days it was obvious that it wasn't something I'd just eaten or indigestion so I went to the doctor's and he gave me . . . he examined me and apparently it was wind, that's all. But it was something I hadn't experienced before that obviously wasn't just indigestion so I felt I ought to go and see him.'

And Mrs R, when her daughter complained of stomach ache over a period of two days, took her to the doctor to rule out potentially serious conditions:

(R35) (Mrs R) 'Alison was complaining of stomach ache for a couple of days, really complaining and I made an appointment and took her to the doctor in case it was appendicitis or something like that. I didn't really think it was but I wanted to make sure.'

As I noted in the previous chapter, the duration of symptoms is often used by the respondents to assert that a condition is severe or trivial irrespective of whether that condition is taken to the doctor. Under the assumption that trivial conditions are of short duration any symptoms that last for a few days or more can be seen to be of a more serious nature. Mrs G used this assumption in deciding that her stomach pains were not an ordinary problem such as indigestion but a complaint that required medical attention. This assumption is frequently used prospectively in mapping future courses of action. At one interview Mrs P's ankles had been swollen and painful for a few days; although she had not been to the doctor, she said, 'You know, if it does continue I obviously will'. When Mr P complained of pain and stiffness in his neck and shoulders it was attributed to draught from driving with the window down and resolved itself without recourse to medical attention. Mrs P, however, went on to say, 'If it had persisted I think possibly he would have gone to the doctor 'cos I said to him, well, you know, if you'd have lifted the children or messing about with them you can hurt yourself without realizing'. Here, persistence of the symptoms would have called for a different explanation and a different strategy of action. This wait and see attitude was presented by some of the respondents as a general strategy they adopted when faced with any problematic experience. Mrs F said, 'If there's anything wrong I ignore it and hope it'll go away and it usually does'. And when I asked Mrs N if the backaches she reported caused her or her husband any problems she said:

(N12) (Mrs N) 'Well, not really. I mean, obviously if it's something that keeps on then we'd go to the doctor. But I think one always waits and waits and then one has to go to the doctor but that applies to anything that you have.'

This general strategy may also be applied to specific symptom episodes and a period of time may be established after which professional attention becomes an appropriate course of action:

(G32) (Mrs G) 'I had this irritation at the opening of my vagina but I gave it a week and it went otherwise I would have gone [to the doctor]. But it was sort of at the end of the week, by Saturday Roger said to me that I ought to go to the doctor's and I said I would go by Monday if it hadn't gone but it had gone.'

In this case the symptoms had disappeared within the time period set and the doctor was not consulted. Not only did the resolution of the symptoms remove the need for professional attention it also meant that a definite explanation of the problem was unnecessary. When I asked her if she knew what had caused the irritation Mrs G said, 'No, not really, I just wondered if it might have been the fact that I'd stopped taking the pill'.

This wait-and-see strategy provides an opportunity to see if the symptoms will resolve themselves or get worse. Mrs S had her breathing problem for two weeks before she went to see the doctor. I asked her what it was that made her decide to go:

(S38) (Mrs S) 'Well, it just got worse, when it got really bad I thought well I must go to the doctor. That first week or so it wasn't bad enough and by the second week . . . and not only that, I was worried. At first I wasn't too worried about it, I thought maybe it's something that'll go away. It didn't so I made an appointment and went to see him.'

Mrs R used a similar procedure in the following account:

(R36) (Mrs R) 'I had an infection in my face which started with what looked like a spot and it spread and spread and eventually as I saw it was just spreading I went to the doctor. I waited a few days because at first I thought it was just a spot which would go away and then I got another one and another one and I ended up with about four. And more recently I got a boil under my arm which I take to be a similar sort of thing. By the time I went to the doctor I realized what it was and realized it wasn't going to get better.'

Both of these accounts contain implicit notions of when it is appropriate to consult a doctor, and these provide the rationale for the initial delay and the subsequent consultation. The delay is accounted for by the fact that the symptoms were first seen to be trivial and likely to resolve themselves. The gradual realization that this was not the case is presented as leading to a redefinition of the situation and the formulation of a new plan of action. Nothing resembling what has been called a critical incident can be detected in these accounts.

The legitimacy of this notion of duration of a problem as an interpretive procedure may be affirmed when it is seen to feature in professional decision-making. If it is used by doctors in planning courses of action then it may reasonably be used by lay actors in determining when and how to act. Mrs P reported taking her daughter to the doctor with bronchitis:

(P19) (Mrs P) 'And, erm, well it took so long to really clear, I was taking her to the doctor every few days for him to sound her chest and he said to me, she'd finished the antibiotic and he said it's at last clearing but if it had gone on we'd have had her chest X-rayed.'

As it happened the bronchitis reappeared a few weeks later and Mrs P, deciding that it had not in fact really cleared asked that they 'get to the root of the problem' and her daughter was referred to hospital for X-ray.

Good reasons for not seeing the doctor

During the course of the interviews the respondents not only provided rationales of why they consulted the doctor about some problems, they also, in response to my questions, offered reasons why on some occasions the problems they described had not been subject to professional attention. The answers they gave to my questions provided them with yet another opportunity for showing that their help-seeking behaviour conformed to the general criteria that defined appropriate consultations.

Given the general statements about visiting the doctor I quoted at the beginning of the chapter the respondents have at hand a ready-made rationale for not seeking professional treatment. That is, they only need assert that an experience falls outside that range of problems for which a visit to the doctor is appropriate. Having established that responsible action consists in visiting the doctor 'only when it's necessary', 'only when I need to' or 'only if it's something serious', failure to consult may be legitimized by defining the problem at hand as trivial or as a condition which does not require expert advice. The latter would consist of a problem that any lay person might be expected to treat:

(R37) (Int.) 'Can you remember any incidents or complaints that you haven't bothered taking to the doctor?'

(Mrs R) 'Lee has had a cold but I didn't take him to the doctor, it wasn't, it didn't warrant it.'

(R38) (Mrs R had told me that she had recently had a migraine.)

(Int.) 'Do you have migraines? I don't remember you mentioning them before.'

(Mrs R) 'I have had them . . . not as well, not a lot. It happens very occasionally. It's never troubled me to any great extent but I have had them. Erm . . . but again I've never done anything about it because it's never been serious enough.'

(R39) (Mrs R had been violently sick one evening in the week prior to an interview.)

(Int.) 'Did you bother going to the doctor's with it?'

(Mrs R) 'Oh no, because I wouldn't have been able to go to the doctor's, I felt far too ill and I wouldn't dream of calling him in for a thing like that because I don't, you know, unless it continues I don't think it merits calling a doctor in and by next morning I was all right.'

In these three examples taken from interviews with Mrs R the character of the problems described is such that professional attention is un-necessary. In the last extract Mrs R distinguishes two routes via which professional attention may be obtained and shows how the nature of the complaint was such that it was ruled out in both. She felt too ill to be able to go and see the doctor and the complaint was not sufficiently severe to justify asking him to make a home visit. Similarly, Mrs P said that her husband had not been to the doctor with his stiff neck because 'It was such a trifling thing to go about probably, you know', and when her son woke up one night with pains in the legs, a complaint which he gets 'now and again', she said 'I haven't had him to the doctor 'cos it's such a spasmodic thing that I've never really bothered much about it, you know'. Mrs G had not consulted the doctor about a sore throat 'because I wouldn't have gone until it got worse than it was' nor had she been about her constipation 'because it's never really upset me'. The respondents not only claimed that they had not been to the doctor because their problems were trivial or inconsequential they legitimated this strategy by invoking professional definitions of the situation:

(G33) (Mrs G had reported in her health diary that she had recently had oral ulcers.)
    (Int.) 'Have you been to see the doctor?'
    (Mrs G) 'Oh no.'
    (Int.) 'Why not?'
    (Mrs G) 'Well, he'd think I'm a nut case, it's so trivial.'

(G34) (Int.) 'If you remember last time [i.e. as reported in health diary] you had a cold you went to get some medicine, why didn't you go to the doctor this time, why didn't you go and see him about it?'
    (Mrs G) 'It's too trivial, a waste of his time, if I could buy something.'
    (Int.) 'Well, why do you think a cold is trivial? What makes a cold trivial?'
    (Mrs G) 'A doctor.'
    (Int.) 'Makes it trivial?'
    (Mrs G) 'Yes, they'd treat it as trivial, if you went with a cold they'd treat it as trivial, they'd treat you as if you were wasting their time. They wouldn't be particularly pleased. I don't know whether he'd say he wasn't pleased but I don't think he'd treat me sympathetically. They haven't got time for people with colds.'

Here, Mrs G is able to demonstrate that her action with regard to various problems is in line with professional conceptions of what is appropriate. These definitions are indicated by the way the doctor is expected to respond to patients who consult with the type of disorders she describes. Although the doctor may not convey these definitions directly, 'I don't know whether he'd say', they can be read by means of their external expression in the way the doctor treats the patient. The conflict between doctor and patient to which this may give rise can be avoided by attempts to conform to professional definitions of the situation. This involves presenting only with complaints that the doctor will view as worthy of his attention. That this strategy is not always successful, however, can be seen by Mrs G's complaint in G28. In constructing this legitimation Mrs G draws on commonsense knowledge about the ways in which doctors typically react to problems of a given type. This is a product of doctors' public statements on the matter (Cartwright 1967), direct experience, and the stories of medical encounters that are a feature of everyday discourse (Stimson and Webb 1976).

Though the criteria of seriousness that doctors are assumed to employ in judging appropriate consulting behaviour may be invoked by patients in legitimating their own actions the definitions that inform doctors' actions are not always acceptable to lay members. Following her telephone call to the doctor in G28 Mrs G was given instructions on how to feed her son and told to take him up to the surgery on the Monday following the Saturday on which the incident occurred:

> (G35) (Mrs G) 'Anyway, he wouldn't come he just took my diagnosis as being correct and that was it. He wouldn't . . . I mean they would never, I mean the only time he would ever come out, you know, to a baby even a baby would be, oh it would have to be something really serious.'

Formulations such as this may be read as complaints, as instances where professional definitions and the practices they inform determine outcomes such as lack of home visits, but where lay definitions should have formed the basis for action. Mrs G clearly regards it as unacceptable that the doctor took her diagnosis as correct rather than make the home visit she thought necessary. However, interactional problems such as this may be invoked to legitimate failure to consult since they are presented as barriers preventing the respondents from acting in ways they think appropriate.

If rational action may be defined as action that serves an actor's purposes or interests, then failure to consult a doctor may be deemed rational if it can be shown that to do so would be in conflict with these purposes or interests. The respondents frequently asserted that they or individuals known to them would suffer pain or discomfort in preference to the consequences they anticipated following from seeing the doctor. Mr P, for example, refused to see the doctor because he was afraid he would be again referred for ECT. In contrast, Mrs R was only too pleased for her husband to be treated as a psychiatric in-patient, despite protests from his family who were worried about the stigma attached to such treatment, because 'my feeling was if he could get better more quickly by going into hospital then please go into hospital immediately'. Mrs R was then able to present her in-laws' response as irrational since their desire to have him treated at home was seen to be designed to protect the family's good name rather than serving the interests of her husband's health.

Mrs P periodically suffered pains from a duodenal ulcer which usually woke her in the middle of the night and continued to be a problem for a week or more. At one interview she described a development of the condition which, contrary to my expectations that this would act as a trigger, she had not taken to the doctor:

(P20) (Mrs P) 'This last time I found that I had the most terrible sort of sensation in my mouth, I felt as if I was almost going to be sick really. I sort of sat on the edge of my bed and thought, gosh, am I going to be sick and I sat there and I thought, oh blimey, not at this time of the night when you're only half with it and then it passed off.'

(Int.) 'And has that happened before, can you remember?'

(Mrs P) 'I don't think it has, no, I can't remember that it has, you know. Usually it's just this terrible gnawing sensation in my stomach and I'll either reach for tablets or something, you know.'

(Int.) 'Did you go and see the doctor this time?'

(Mrs P) 'No, I didn't. Well, as I say, it's just that I've got the things, I know sort of what to do really. I mean if I went whether he'd send me for a barium meal or again, I don't know, erm, because I had all those originally you know and they're not exactly something I relish the thought of again because when it is troubling you like that you see if you're going to have a barium meal you have to go for hours without any food and the pain builds up and it gets really grim, you know. I'm not being funny, it's utter misery and so as I sort of know what to do really I sort of do it and after a week or so it starts to die down and fades out completely.'

Past experience had taught Mrs P a routine that could be used to manage the pains from her ulcer relatively successfully. In general this meant that it was usually unnecessary for her to see the doctor because she knew exactly what to do. Her reason for avoiding going back with this new developoment resides in her evaluation of the likely consequences of such a consultation. The diagnostic procedures involved, because they require a radical alteration in her management routine, cause her considerable discomfort. One of her methods of pain control, and incidentally one of the methods she used to prevent the problem occurring in the first place, was to make sure that she did not go for long periods of time without food while one of the requirements of the anticipated diagnostic procedure was that the patient did not eat for several hours. Respondents who had developed routines for dealing with recurring problems of this kind sometimes claimed that they had been to see the doctor following the breakdown of their routine. It does then seem feasible that Mrs P would have viewed this new development differently had it threatened the success of her normal management of the problem.

Using a similar rationale, Mrs R had avoided returning to the doctor with pain in her maxillary sinus because she feared it would necessitate another operation. A year prior to the first interview she had had the root of a tooth removed from the sinus where it had caused an infection. The operation was not entirely successful and she had been warned that it might have to be repeated. However, Mrs R preferred to tolerate the discomfort although occasionally it became quite painful. 'I feel if I go, if I really go back and pursue the matter it will probably necessitate another operation which I want to avoid if I can.' Presumably, Mrs R would accept another operation if the pain became frequent or severe: 'it doesn't happen very often, I don't feel it warrants going back to repeat the whole process.'[5]

In the general statements quoted in the early part of the chapter children were regarded as occupying a special status with regard to deciding whether or not to visit the doctor. Whereas a problem in an adult may be ignored, with a child 'you wouldn't take any chances' or 'you'd be more careful'. The failure to take a child for medical attention thus calls for justification if the public presentation of responsible parenthood is to be maintained. Mrs P and Mrs R invoked versions of the conflict of interests rationale to account for failure to consult the doctor about their children. Following a course of treatment for bronchitis, Mrs P reported that her daughter started coughing 'badly again and at nights' and that she had treated this herself with medicine previously supplied by the doctor:

> (P21) (Mrs P) 'She still sounds wheezy but I haven't taken her so far, but I'm sort of keeping an eye. Well, you know, you sort of feel it's such a nuisance really for the kid herself to keep backwards and forwards, you know, and I'm not keen on too much antibiotic in massive doses, I sort of feel that they'll, you know, it won't have the desired effect if she keeps on she'll get sort of immune, won't she?'

And Mrs R reporting that she had not taken her son to the doctor although she thought he was likely to get an ear infection said, 'I don't want him to spend half his life at the doctor's'. Mothers may also disregard doctor's orders on the grounds that the consequences of following those orders are not in a child's best interests. Mrs P stopped giving her daughter anti-histamines which had been prescribed for an allergy because she thought it was responsible for drying out her nose, making it bleed quite severely.

Rational action is not merely action which serves an individual's interests. As McHugh (1968) suggests, members frequently assert that some means are more efficient than others in achieving certain ends, and characterize behaviour as appropriate or inappropriate depending upon how it facilitates those objectives. Rational action is technically efficient action. Members may then legitimate courses of action by pointing to their viability in bringing about desired ends. Conversely, they may legitimate the non-performance of certain actions on the grounds that they are irrelevant to the attainment of their objectives. One good reason for not going to the doctor is that the cognitive and material resources at his disposal are ineffective in bringing about the resolution of a given problem. Mrs G had not been to the doctor with a cold because 'there's not a great deal he can do for me, is there?' And when Mrs R's daughter caught chicken pox she phoned the doctor and told him but 'didn't bother to take her up there because there's nothing he can do'. Mrs F used a similar rationale to explain why she hadn't been to the doctor when her eyes were swollen with what she assumed was an allergy:

(F24)   (Mrs F) 'I've had . . . I . . . this is something which I get fairly regularly, my eyes get all puffy and it happens about this time of the year, so we, the doctor and I assume that it's all connected with the hay fever which I don't get any more, but it does affect my eyes. This one particularly has been itchy and all sort of swollen but I haven't bothered to go to him because in the past I've been to . . . I've had all the tests that you can think of for what I'm supposed to be allergic to at the allergy clinic and the doctor said he'd met his Waterloo. Another time when my eyes were particularly puffy I went to the hospital and they gave me some cream and I've still got a tiny bit in the tube so I shall put that on and hope it goes away. But, as I say, I don't feel it's worth going to the doctor for because he doesn't know what to give me.'

At a subsequent interview Mrs F reported that following a prolonged episode of the allergy she had been to the doctor who had suggested referral to a specialist:

(F25)   (Mrs F) 'Quite honestly, I don't think I shall bother, I think it's a waste of time because I've been through the pipeline before. I went through one pipeline to a specialist, an eye specialist, and he didn't put his finger on anything and another time I went and had all the allergy tests, I took all my make-up and I had bits of plaster all over my back with all their little bottles they tried and I wasn't allergic to anything except the plaster they stuck them all on with and the doctor said I've met my Waterloo, go home and live with it. So I really don't think there's an awful lot of point going through that lot again.'

Past experience had shown Mrs F that neither the GP nor the specialists to whom she had been referred had been successful in treating what was supposed to be an allergy. Because they were unable to identify any substance to which she was allergic they were unable to formulate effective remedial action. Consequently, going to the doctor about this problem was pointless and a waste of time because it produced no better results than Mrs F's own method of managing the problem.

As I described in Chapter 5 women may invoke the obligations imposed on them by their occupancy of the roles of wife and mother to manage the discrepancy between a definition of illness and the non-performance of illness-relevant behaviours. The same rationale may be invoked to account for failure to go to the doctor. Mrs S, for example, had not been back to see the doctor although the tablets he prescribed for her breathing problem didn't seem to work:

(S39)   (Mrs S) 'I keep saying I will go back but I never have. It's just getting there, you know, finding time in between. I was going to go back when I'd finished the tablets, you know, and say to him, well I've taken them and I don't really feel much better, erm, you know, what do you think now, but, erm, I haven't really had the time to go up there.'

Later in the interview Mrs S provided a detailed description of how her responsibilities as a mother prevented her from finding the time to make an appointment and from getting to see the doctor:

(S40)   (Mrs S) 'I find it's far more difficult to even find time sometimes, say in the morning, I find that the best time to ring up is half-past eight in the morning and then you can make sure of getting through immediately because after that the phone is permanently engaged. Well, I haven't got time when I'm getting the children ready for school to keep trying to ring the doctor up so it's impossible. Sometimes I might think to myself I ought to make an appointment to go and see the doctor and I haven't got the time honestly, it's impossible. And then after the children have gone to school it's either too late and the phone's permanently engaged or it's too late to make an appointment for that day. I don't know what's going to be happening the following day so really it's very difficult. I can't go up in the evenings because the children they come home from school so I think it's half of the thing why I don't always get in touch with the doctor. Once again it's the time factor as far as I'm concerned. And then again in the holidays when I'm not rushing it means traipsing the children up there. I prefer to go without if it's for me. If it's a child, obviously it's a different thing, you've got to take them anyway.'

Mrs S presents her duties as a mother as a barrier preventing her gaining access to the doctor because these conflict with certain features of the way access to the doctor is organized. At one interview Mrs P described how she had been unable to go into hospital for tests because of her responsibilities as a mother:

> (P22) (Mrs P) 'Some years ago I had these very bad heads and I was under a doctor at the hospital and I had X-rays, head X-rays from all angles and also a chest X-ray and they never discovered anything. They said they would have liked me to go in for further tests but they realized that the children were young at the time and it wasn't very convenient for me to go in.'

Entry into medical care may be viewed as desirable (Mrs S, for example, recognized that she ought to go back to the doctor about her breathing problem) but may not occur because of constraints imposed upon the individual. That constraints such as role responsibilities are legitimate barriers to seeing the doctor can only be seen if reference is made to knowledge about the role concerned and typical ways in which it is performed. Mothers are expected to put the interests of their children before their own and in so doing may be identified as good mothers. Consequently, they cannot be identified as irresponsible in failing to find time to seek medical help. There seemed to be a consensus of opinion between Mrs P and her doctors that her duties as a mother came before the investigations they would have liked to have performed. In defining the outcome as consensus opinion Mrs P underlines the fact that her choice of action was socially and professionally sanctioned. As a result, her action is difficult to fault.

Interactional and organizational barriers to seeing the doctor

In the account given by Mrs S above, she not only refers to the way in which her responsibilities as a mother create difficulties in gaining access to medical care, she also cites the way in which access is organized as a contributory source of problems. During the course of the interviews the respondents described a variety of interactional and organizational barriers which they claimed had an influence on their help-seeking behaviour. The extent to which these problems did prevent them from seeing the doctor is, given the methodological approach, problematic. I prefer to take the view that our discussions of illness behaviour provided them with opportunities to construct complaints about doctors and medical practice. Consequently, their identification of these barriers shifted the responsibility for their failure to seek professional help to those involved in the provision of medical care.

The interactional problems experienced in consultations that the respondents described consisted of the ways in which doctors deliberately or unwittingly challenged their competence or otherwise failed to conform to their definitions of the situation. In the case presented at the beginning of the chapter Mrs G interpreted the doctor's response to the telephone call about her son as an attempt to fault the appropriateness of her actions. As a result, she reports being 'put off' the doctor. Mrs G continued her account by formulating a further complaint:

(G36) (Mrs G) 'I was told to take him up to the surgery on the Monday morning. Even then, it put me off that. I took him then and he was all wrapped up because it was a freezing cold morning and he said, he said to Daniel and what are you going to wear when the winter comes, you know?'

In any encounter, statements by one party may be read by the other as criticisms or attempts to fault performance. I take it that the statement by the doctor to Mrs G's son was read by her as a challenge to her competence. One formulation of the statement as such a challenge would be to read it as a claim that the child was over-dressed and, by implication, Mrs G an over-protective mother. Mrs G, however, provides for her own competence and the relevance of her actions when she says 'it was a freezing cold day'.

That there is a power differential in doctor-patient interactions whereby the doctor, because of his control of cognitive and material resources, is able to impose his definitions of the situation on the patient and comment on their rationality has often been described in the sociological literature on the doctor-patient relationship. That the reverse is more difficult because of the imbalance of power has also been recognized. Patients are also aware that there is a power differential in the relationship so that they are relatively disadvantaged. As Mrs F remarked when a doctor diagnosed and treated her eye problem as an infection although she knew it was an allergy, 'I knew it was an allergy but he insisted it was an infection, but you can't argue, can you?' And Mrs R commenting on a visit during her second pregnancy to the endocrinologist who had prescribed corticosteroids for the first said, 'He said haven't you been taking it all along and I said no, whatever for, and he said, oh I would have expected you to take it all the time and, er . . . I didn't argue with him, a very well-known man who's not to be argued with'.

These kind of conflicts, usually covert, that may occur when patients consult doctors, may be invoked by patients as constraints on entering into consultations. At the same time they present strategies that they claim to use to influence the doctor's evaluation of them and the appropriateness of their consultation and thereby minimize conflict:

(G37) (Mrs G) 'The next time I went up because Daniel had got a very bad cold. I was reluctant to go because of the way that he'd treated me the first time and sort of when I went in I made it sort of quite obvious, I said to him, well I thought I'd better come up now rather than have you out in the middle of the night. I didn't think, you know, that you'd find that very pleasant.'

Stimson and Webb (1976) have suggested that patients' accounts of their encounters with doctors are formulated in such a way that the activity and integrity of the patient are stressed and the inequality between the doctor and patient is redressed. They also suggest that the reconstruction of the encounters depends as much on the shared opinions and assumptions of the teller and the audience about the social world of doctors and patients as it does on the recall of the details of the original exchange. In this account Mrs G presents herself as managing the encounter with a doctor who in the past had proved difficult by offering a good reason for her visit at the opening of their interaction. Stimson and Webb would probably claim that it is unlikely that the encounter happened in the way the respondent describes. However, irrespective of the way in which an observer would have characterized the scene, Mrs G must present an account in a way that makes it clear what she was up to. That is, a listener or reader must be able to make sense of what she claims to have done in the situation in which she claims to have done it. I take it that her statement at the opening of their encounter was an attempt to influence the doctor's definition of the appropriateness of her visit for a disorder that might otherwise be characterized as trivial. One reading of what she claims to have said is that it is preferable from the doctor's point of view for her to consult with a complaint that might be relatively trivial rather than wait for her son's condition to deteriorate, which might have involved the doctor in a night call. To the extent that strategies of this kind are employed by patients, they are made necessary by the ambiguity with which many disorders present. Lay knowledge is not always sufficient to allow an unambiguous definition to be constructed. Mothers then may often decide to err on the side of caution. They are also necessitated by the patient's awareness, either derived from direct experience or indirectly from the accounts of others, of the way in which doctors may respond to consultations they see as unnecessary. Mrs P, unsure of whether or not to consult the doctor when her daughter began coughing again following the completion of a course of antibiotics, left the decision to the doctor:

> (P23) (Mrs P) 'Over the week-end she's been coughing a lot and I thought, I don't know, she sounds really rattly there again and I phoned the doctor on the Monday and I said I don't want to bring her up if you don't think it's necessary but I said she does sound rather wheezy on her chest again. Oh, he said, bring her up.'

Another way in which doctors are seen to challenge patients' competence is their refusal to impart information. Mrs S and Mrs R complained about the difficulty of finding out what is going on:

(S41) (Mrs S) 'I'm so worried about Michael going to hospital for his next check-up. I know it's stupid but I just tremble now I can feel myself just going all funny, you know. It's stupid, he's doing so well now but I just can't help myself. Mr B I think as much as anything, he frightens me to death. He's the surgeon, he did the operation. Well, I mean he's a very good surgeon, he's marvellous but it's just . . . when we first went up there I suppose they did it for about six weeks and we thought six weeks that's not too bad and it turned out to be six months. I mean, it's a heck of a difference from six weeks. And I felt oh I think that's rotten saying things like that, I'd rather be told the truth from the beginning, you know, if they say it's going to be six months you accept it but from six weeks suddenly to go into that long time that annoyed me tremendously. I thought, well, what do they think us parents are, sort of thing, you know, I'd rather be told the truth about things. This is what I think is wrong with doctors they don't tell you anything, I think they think you're a load of kids or something and can't accept the truth so it does make me feel nervous about it.'

(R40) (Mrs R) 'I do feel there is a lack of information given. It's very much up to the individual doctor, some doctors will discuss fully whatever it is wrong with you and others won't. I feel our present practice don't discuss fully enough although I must make one exception when my husband went to Dr M he did discuss the thing with us very freely but, erm, at other times I think he doesn't, I think he tends to treat the patient as a bit of an idiot who's not going to understand anyway, I think this is quite general to a lot of doctors, you know, don't bother to tell them 'cos they're not going to understand, just give them their prescription and they can go away like good children and take it which I object to very strongly.'

In both of these cases part of the respondent's indignation stems from the way in which doctors are assumed to characterize patients. It is the doctor's view of patients as 'children' or 'idiots' incapable of understanding what is wrong with them or accepting the truth that is seen to underlie their reluctance to discuss matters fully or otherwise give an accurate picture of the situation.[6] That doctors see patients in such terms is a source of annoyance since it defines them as incompetents and challenges their taken-for-granted status as responsible adults. It is not without its other consequences. Mrs S claimed that part of her nervous problem prior to hospital visits originated in this lack of information and Mrs R went on to describe the effects of ignorance:

(R41) (Mrs R) 'If you don't know you worry about it, or at least I do, if I know what's happening I can say right well, you know, I, this, that and the other, but if I don't know then I start thinking well I wonder what's wrong and I wonder what I'm taking and I wonder what effect it can have and I do start worrying although I don't generally worry much about my health. I don't like the unknown and, er, I can get very indignant about it because then I feel very unhappy, once it's explained to me then I'm much more at ease about it.'

In this extract Mrs R reaffirms a point I made at the beginning of Chapter 4. Without the relevant knowledge at her disposal she is unable to achieve a sense of order and is, consequently, unhappy. Given that the problem is presented in this way it suggests a rational course of action. 'I always ask, I mean I just insist and if they don't explain I just go on asking or I'll ask the chemist who's prescribing as well so that I know what I'm taking.' That this contravenes what Mrs R imagines is a doctor's conception of a good patient is recognized when she says, 'I must be a doctor's nightmare'. That this is a typical experience of patients was indicated by Mrs S when she said, 'It happens to the majority [of people she knew], they just don't tell you anything'.

Doctors were also seen to challenge the respondent's competence by not acquiescing to patients' defined needs. Mrs G, for example, told me that she had a long history of tonsillitis and past experience had taught her its typical course and the most efficient way of managing it:

(G38) (Mrs G) 'Well, sometimes it starts off as a cold. This has, you know, been the only thing that I've ever suffered with, I've ever gone to the doctor's with, my medical card's just covered with sore throats and tonsillitis from when I was about seven or eight until now. Perhaps starts as a cold and then I just get a sore throat and it, if I don't go and get some antibiotics from the doctor, it turns into tonsillitis. So when I've had a sore throat, rather than let it get hold of me, I'd say go up there I'd go to the doctor's and ask him if he'd give me some penicillin or some kind of antibiotic because I knew that if I took them it would go within a matter of a couple of days, but if I'd waited say a week and then went it would have got hold of me and I'd have to have a fortnight at home off work. And I went a couple of times like that and he sort of, I mean he gave it to me but he was er . . . I don't know, a bit annoyed.'

Mrs G had a proven recipe at hand for dealing with sore throats which was designed to prevent it turning into tonsillitis with consequent absence from work. That involved presenting early on in its course and requesting antibiotics from the doctor. The doctor is presented as defining the situation differently; although he granted Mrs G's request he was perceived to be 'a bit annoyed'. That Mrs G's strategy was a reasonable one is given by its technical efficiency:

(G39) (Mrs G) 'And yet it did, you know, that was true, that within, I didn't have any time off in those eighteen months, I didn't have a day off at all. And yet I could probably have had a month off with those couple of bad throats.'

Mrs F reported how both she and her daughter had experienced problems when they went to one doctor for the renewal of their prescriptions for the pill:

(F26) (Mrs F) 'There's something about some of these doctors, one really put my back up and, you know, I'm quite a sort of mild person, he really upset me and he upset my daughter who went for the pill. OK, so he was anti-pill but it's there and it's available and . . . I don't know, the argument seemed to be, what at your age, at my advanced age, I went to him in the January and I was forty-six and I was only just forty-six, the attitude was you're forty-seven you should be thinking about facing, you know, old age and the rest of it embracing, you know . . .'
    (Int.) 'Mm.'
    (Mrs F) 'the menopause, what do you want with the pill at forty-seven, and I said to him mildly, forty-six, and anyway he managed to bring back into the conversation forty-seven again, you see, and anyway he then gives it me for six months and then he says you've got to think about giving up and I thought I'm damned if I'm seeing you again mate so I made quite sure I went on a morning when Dr M was there . . .'
    (Int.) 'Yes.'
    (Mrs F) '. . . and the attitude was so different. I said, you know, almost apologetically, please may I have another and he said, well, of course, we don't want you pregnant at thirty-two, do we? Now what a different attitude, totally different and as I say he upset my daughter so much that she left the place in floods of tears and went straight to another doctor and said can I come as a private patient and he said, yes.'
    (Int.) 'Did he refuse to give her a prescription?'
    (Mrs F) 'No, he didn't really, but he was going to argue about it and he wanted her to have a smear test which she thought was somewhat unnecessary at the age of seventeen and he insists, you know, that she has this smear test and she said, well, Dr Z or Dr M have never gone into this at my age . . . at my age, OK, but I don't think it's necessary at her age and there was an attitude that, er, he said, well perhaps you think I want to look at you undressed or something, you know.'

In both of the instances described by Mrs F the doctor is seen to be imposing his definition of the situation on Mrs F and her daughter, a definition which conflicts with their own self-perceived needs. The account is constructed in such a way that the doctor's attitude may be interpreted as unreasonable, evidence of an underlying 'anti-pill' stance, rather than the alternative formulation that he was practising good medicine. Given this perceived underlying attitude the doctor's specific recommendations may be taken to be attempts on his part to erect barriers preventing access to the goods and services they desire. Advising Mrs F to think about giving up the pill and recommending that her daughter have a smear test may fall within what is medically defined as good practice, serving the interests of the patient. However, that these actions are to be read as evidence of the doctor being unreasonably difficult in the consultation is given by the facts that Mrs F presents. The doctor's definition of Mrs F as too old is a product of his consistent and deliberate over-estimation of her age. This, and his general attitude, are contrasted with that of Dr M who not only under-estimates her age but willingly prescribes the pill. The doctor's insistence that Mrs F's daughter have a smear test is also to be seen to be unreasonable given her age and given the fact that two other doctors have never thought it necessary that she submit to these investigations. Mrs F and her daughter managed these difficult interactions by avoiding that doctor in the future.

In a subsequent interview Mrs F described recent changes in her doctor's practice that had changed the nature of medical care and created barriers between doctor and patient. This was invoked as an influence on when she would choose a consultation as the way of dealing with certain problems:

(F27)   (Mrs F) 'I think somehow we look on the doctor more or less as a last resort. I mean for other people I always say go, but if it's for me I think ignore it, it'll go away. You know, somehow it's too much . . . I don't know . . . it's not the same going to the doctor as it used to be. It somehow used to be a pleasure. When Dr M was on his own and we all knew him really well and he had this one receptionist who was a sweet woman and lived on the premises we really felt we were one of his family. And it's the same with everything these days, everything expands, there are now three of them practising there you know you never know who you're going to see and when you go he's got three receptionists and it seems to me they are there to stop you seeing him if possible. They want to know what your symptoms are when you phone up and if they don't think you're ill you don't get transferred to the doctor, you don't get an appointment, you know, they . . . I'm resentful somehow over doctors and their practices. I'm just a number, just an address on a card. I'm not me any more that the doctor knows and the receptionist knows. This is basically why under the old set-up I would have gone to Dr M and said, well, look my eyes have come up again this year, anything fresh we can try? But now as I say there are three receptionists to get past first and then you're lucky to see who you want to see. Erm, this is something I don't want to know about, I'd rather stay away unless it's really desperate.'

For Mrs F the essence of good medical practice involves personal knowledge of the patient and his family. Recent changes in the way the practice is organized, its expansion to three doctors, and the introduction of receptionists, have resulted in an impersonal service in which the doctor no longer knows his patients as individuals. In addition, the function of the receptionists appears to be one of keeping patients from seeing the doctor since they, by their control of the appointment book, are able to question the appropriateness of the patient's decision to see the doctor and impose their own judgements where they think necessary. The problems involved in negotiating access and the patients' lack of control over outcome in terms of which doctor they see are presented by Mrs F as sufficient reasons for staying away from the doctor 'unless it's really desperate'.

That the system is impersonal and prevents the exercise of knowledge of the patient by those involved in controlling access, which would otherwise allow them to make adequate judgements about the appro- priateness of requests for consultations or home visits, is evidenced by the case Mrs F described and which I presented in Chapter 5 (extract F17). When her husband had flu Mrs F telephoned the practice to request a home visit and 'all I got was the receptionist fending me off'. Had the system involved the exercise of personal knowledge those controlling access 'would have known this man must be ill if he's asking for a doctor because he's never been near us, never bothered us' and would then have been in a position to make an adequate decision. While this would have been possible under the old set-up, under the new set-up 'who knows the individual any more?'

Experiences such as this lead to the conclusion that the practice no longer cares, 'who cares any more?', and may then act as a legitimation for not visiting the doctor when it might have otherwise been thought necessary. Just prior to the last interview with his wife, Mr F had a very bad cold and a temperature and had to stay in bed for two days. When I asked Mrs F why she had not had the doctor round to see him she said, 'Well, because last time he had flu the doctor didn't want to know. I went round and I was given a piece of paper how to treat influenza so as far as I'm concerned, you know, that's it. I've gone off doctors, I have really, I'm very disillusioned'.

Similar points were made by Mrs S in discussing the difficulties of getting appointments with the doctor of her choice:

(S42) (Mrs S) 'Actually it's a hell of a job trying to get an appointment always, you know, with him because Dr M is pretty busy up there and I do like to see him rather than any others 'cos I've known him since I was eleven years old, you know, as far as I'm concerned he's my doctor, he knows me, he knows what makes me tick and sometimes you phone through and the receptionists are, you know, stupid. You try, it's ridiculous, you know, you'd think they were Mafia or something trying to get past to see Dr M and it's so stupid and I get mad. You know, I think who the hell are they to talk to me like that? I know they have a certain amount of job to do but they're like little Hitlers and that's another thing that puts me off.'

(Int.) 'You always ask to see Dr M?'

(Mrs S) 'Yes, he knows me, er, I must say I don't know if Dr Z's even there any more, somebody said he'd retired, now I liked him he's very nice but he just didn't seem to know me and there's another little man up there I've only seen Dr S, I've only seen him once a long time ago and he was very nice but once again I just felt that they didn't know me. Dr M is very good and he's very kind, you know, he's very good. He knows I have Michael, he understands my problems so therefore I like to see him and if I can get an appointment with him then I'm happy. If I can't get one the same day I'll wait for him. The thing is, you see, the receptionist probably thinks why sort of thing when there's other doctors, but obviously they don't know that I've been going to see him for, you know, I just feel it's as if, well, that's it, I want to go and see Dr M. They do put you off though some of these women, they're ogres they really are and I'm not the only one to say that, the majority of people do. It's most off-putting really, I don't think they have a right to talk to people the way they do talk to them.'

(Int.) 'Yes.'

(Mrs S) 'One lady up there, she's very nice. If I ring in a morning sometimes I get her but she doesn't always answer the phone. But there is another, she's most unpleasant and it puts me off, otherwise I might, you know, have made my appointment sooner.'

Because they do not know her history and her relationship with Dr M, the receptionists are not in a position to understand her desire to see only him; they 'probably think why when there's other doctors'. Like Mrs F, Mrs S invokes the problems involved in gaining access as a good reason for delaying visiting the doctor or avoiding seeing him at all. If she were not 'put off' by the receptionists who she sees as having no right to talk to her in the way that they do, she claims she would already have made an appointment to see the doctor about her breathing problem. Because of the difficulties of negotiating access to the doctor of her choice Mrs S chose to take care of most disorders herself:

(S43) (Mrs S) 'If I ring through and say to them I'd like to make an appointment to see Dr M, I'll probably get one of them saying you can't see him, he's not here or something like this, you know. So if I can we dose ourselves up unless it's really urgent and if I think it is then I'll have to go and see him. But if I could look after everything myself then I'd do that. It's much quicker and much easier and no bad results yet, everything's, you know, sorted itself out.'

That these barriers were seen by Mrs S as the product of the actions of the receptionists rather than the doctors is evident in the following account:

(S44) (Mrs S) 'This is a thing that'll give you an idea. I pulled a muscle in my neck just at the back here and I went to Dr Z and he gave me a pain killer, Distalgesic I think it was. I started taking them and they were good so I finished those and I had about four left and I thought well I'll phone through rather than come out 'cos it's a bit difficult getting out sometimes, you know, so I phoned through and oh I'm sorry Mrs S, it was this dreadful one again, we don't take prescriptions on the phone any more, you'll have to come up and get it, you see, but this once she said this once we'll, she was going to do me a favour, we'll make up the prescription for you and, erm, mustn't do it any more, you just feel like a child . . .'

(Int.) 'Yes.'

(Mrs S) 'you know, and this is the sort of thing that gets me, so I said oh I'm sorry I won't do it again, you know, and that was it. So I went up there and Dr M was in and he was so nice you know, although she was there he said, oh hello, Shirley, you know, it's been Shirley . . .'

(Int.) 'Yes.'

(Mrs S) 'you know, and it's so nice, well how are you and what have you been doing? I've got your prescription here, do you want to come in and collect it and he signed it for me and there was no comment from him, well I shouldn't have gone up, I shouldn't have phoned through and all the rest of it and it just makes you wonder if it's just them lot that say it. But there you are, I got my tablets, he didn't query it, he didn't even, you know, worry that I was getting them and not coming up to see him.'

In contrasting the responses of the receptionist and the doctor, Mrs S demonstrates that her request for a repeat prescription was not unreasonable. The doctor is certainly presented as being happy to accept that state of affairs and willingly granted Mrs S's request. Consequently, it may be concluded that the receptionist was not acting on the doctor's authority, 'it just makes you wonder if it's them lot that say it'. This absolves the doctor from any responsibility for the presence of this particular barrier, for it is the receptionist alone who is seen to be at fault.

The respondents not only presented receptionists as routinely questioning the necessity of a visit to the doctor, they also described some of the methods they used in persuading the receptionists that an appointment was necessary. This largely consisted of invoking features of the case concerned to demonstrate the severity of the problem. In Chapter 4 I described how Mrs G and Mrs S reported instances in which the age of children was invoked when receptionists queried whether there was any need for the doctor to be seen. Mrs P described how she had gone up to the surgery with her husband only to find that there had been a mistake in the appointment and he had been incorrectly booked in for the next day. 'So I explained, well look he really does feel ill, he's got up out of bed to come, isn't there a chance that the doctor will see him?' And when she telephoned the surgery to request a home visit for her daughter the receptionist said ' "Can't you bring her up?" and I said not with a temperature of 104'. Here the respondents attempt to trade on commonsense knowledge that they assume the receptionists will use in deciding how to allocate the doctor's time. In attempting to demonstrate the severity of the problem in this way they assume the receptionist will see the sense of the matter and grant their requests. Where this does not happen the respondents report being annoyed and disillusioned. They also clearly resent the fact that barriers such as this exist, which require time and energy to negotiate. These barriers constitute an organizational challenge to patients' competence to decide when it is necessary to see the doctor. Respondents' accounts are then critiques of the organization of medical practice and a reaffirmation of their competence and rationality.

Alternatives to seeing the doctor

As numerous social and epidemiological surveys have shown, the majority of symptom episodes are managed independently of formal medical agencies. Where doctors are not consulted, or where professional attention fails to produce a satisfactory outcome, individuals resort to alternative methods of coping with the disorders that arise. The options available for them to pursue are fairly limited: they may do nothing, they may self-medicate, or they may consult one or more non-licensed practitioners such as chemists or spiritualists. Where disorders are recurrent, individuals may develop routine ways of dealing with them without recourse to professional attention. These routines may be developed in consultation with doctors who provide the cognitive and material resources on which the routine is based, or they may develop routines through self-experimentation. The extent to which such routines can be developed and maintained independently of doctors depends upon whether the resources a doctor controls are necessary to the routine. As Mrs G said, 'In this country you can't obtain antibiotics can you and that kind of thing so therefore you've got to go to the doctor in order to, if it's something that needs that kind of treatment then you've got to in order to get them, haven't you?'

The routines that the respondents constructed and employed involved a recipe for action that in the past had proved successful and was assumed would be successful in the future, and a notion of the typical course of a problem which defined what action was to be taken at what time. As I have shown, these notions of the typical course of a problem were also employed in characterizing any particular occurrence of it as severe or otherwise. Departures from this typical course may then be offered as the rationale for new methods of management, or they may call for re-interpretations, such that the problem is no longer seen to be an instance of what it was originally supposed to be.

Management routines may be legitimated as professional constructs or derive their legitimacy from their ability to produce successful outcomes. Mrs S, whose daughter had 'funny tonsils' that troubled her from time to time, described a management routine the doctor recommended she use while judgement on how to resolve the problem was deferred.

(S45) (Mrs S) 'We'll see what we're going to do about them later on when she gets a bit older. But, er . . . I give her a couple of Junior Disprins every so often, you know, and it goes and she's all right. I've taken her temperature, I never had one but I went to Dr Z when Dr M was away and he gave me a thermometer because I'd never had one in the house before, you know, and I took her temperature and it was a bit high and he said every time it happens I should take her temperature and just give her Junior Disprin and don't do anything more than that.'

Mrs P and Mrs F both described routines for managing problems which, while not recommended by the doctor, depended upon material resources supplied by him:

(P24) (Mrs P suffered periodically with pain from a duodenal ulcer.)

(Mrs P) 'Er, usually it'll wake me in the middle of the night or something like that, er, the only way I can describe it is as if some-thing's eating my inside away and I usually have to get up although sometimes I take a glass of milk and some plain biscuits up to bed with me. I've got Nulacin tablets which the doctor gave me and I always keep some of those handy, you know, to suck . . . if I suck one or sometimes two if it's been bad as I'm sort of dropping off to sleep and they sort of dissolve in my mouth through the night that keeps it down 'cos I presume they coat your stomach and that gives it something to work on, you know . . .'

(Int.) 'Mm.'

(Mrs P) 'through the night hours. But, erm, I did have a bit of a bad spell this last time, you know, it was rather uncomfortable but, er, I know what I've got to do when it does flare up so I just sort of plod on, you know. The thing is you see, never to go without food, something inside, erm, if I'm going shopping and I sort of stop and think now it's some time since I had breakfast or something, I'll have something quick before I go out because I know it's fatal once I get that terribly empty feeling because it starts paining again, you see, so the thing is to keep having something every couple of hours and then I'm OK.'

(Int.) 'Did the doctor advise you to do that sort of . . .?'

(Mrs P) 'Well, erm, not exactly, but the thing is my brother along the road, he had ulcer trouble for years and eventually he had the operation and he said I wish I'd had it years ago 'cos now of course he can eat everything and anything. But I don't watch what I eat, perhaps I should but, as I say, it doesn't flare up all that often and so, you know, I go merrily on. But if I have trouble with it, you know, I'm very, very careful.'

(F28) (Mrs F) 'I do get allergies, my eyes swell, my face swells. I take antihistamines for most of the summer. There again it doesn't necessitate a visit, just a phone call for a prescription 'cos I know what I need. I just take an occasional Piriton in case it's an allergy and I use a little bit of the cream I was given at the hospital which I have left and it seems to keep it down until the season or whatever it is affecting me goes away, you know, it'll probably be for only a few weeks and I shall be all right. I'm sure it'll go away on its own without having to go to the doctor.'

In both of these cases, Mrs P and Mrs F had acquired a body of knowledge about problems which occurred periodically and had developed routines for dealing with them. Mrs P's method of managing the pain from her ulcer involved diet control and the use of drugs previously supplied by the doctor. The control of diet derived from her knowledge of the consequences of going without food for any period of time. Because her brother had suffered from a similar problem she was able to draw on his experience as a resource in understanding and dealing with her own. Mrs F had not been provided with a medically defined method of management but had learnt through experience how to treat what she supposed was an allergy. Her management routine involved taking anti-allergic drugs 'in case it's an allergy' and using cream that she was prescribed on one of her visits to a specialist. Because they knew what to do and had the resources to do it these routines constituted feasible alternatives to visiting the doctor. At subsequent interviews both of these respondents reported that they had recently been to the doctor because their methods of management had broken down. At one interview Mrs F said, 'I've run out of the ointment so I don't know what I shall do' and at the next interview she explained why she had recently been back to the doctor, 'Well, I didn't have any cream left and I didn't have any antihistamines so I more or less had to go'. And Mrs P said, 'This time I went to the doctor because I didn't have the sort of tablet, you know, the Nulacin and he gave me those'.

Where conditions have been treated in the past by a doctor, individuals may acquire resources which may be used in the future given any recurrence of the problem. This may take the form of self-medication with medically prescribed drugs. When Mrs S pulled a muscle in her neck she took some of the tablets she had previously been prescribed. 'The first time I went to see the doctor he gave me these pain killers and he said take those and I had some left and I've been taking them for my neck and it's much better.' Similarly, having been prescribed drugs for her nerves she had the resources at hand for dealing with any future problem herself. 'If I start feeling depressed again I have got some tablets which the doctor gave me last time and I went and I only took a few and I've got them so I'll take them.' Experience of what has proved effective in the past is used to construct future courses of action under the assumption that it will again prove to be effective. At another interview Mrs S was able to use this assumption and knowledge of the typical outcomes to plan alternative methods of dealing with a problem:

> (S46) (Mrs S) 'I've got a headache now but I suppose that's because I've been rushing around. But that will go. I won't take anything for it unless it gets nasty. I find that now I'm having a bit of a sit down it will probably go and if I find it doesn't, I'll take an aspirin and probably in about half an hour it's gone.'

Knowledge about the typical pattern of onset of a disorder may also be used as the basis for preventive action. Mrs R's son suffered fairly frequently with ear trouble and just prior to the first interview he had been to the doctor several times with infections. Because these ear infections had been seen to follow coughs and colds they were the signal for Mrs R to act:

> (R42) (Mrs R) 'He's got a cold at the moment and then we're a little bit careful with him in case he gets an ear infection, you know, we dress him up warmly and that sort of thing which is about all you can do, I think.'

Similarly, Mrs P said of her daughter, 'She might say, oh, my throat hurts and I immediately look and get her to stick her tongue out so I can look down her throat and if there is any inflammation there I usually straight away . . . I don't hang about knowing the throat is troublesome with her'.

The management routines that the respondents reported do not only break down as a result of a lack of the material resources involved, they may also prove to be ineffective following changes in the nature of the problematic experience. That is, a departure from the course a disorder typically takes may call for new interpretations and courses of action. Mrs F, for example, usually ignored the rheumatism that occasionally affected her arm but did go to the doctor once 'when it was particularly painful'. When Mrs R got a headache she didn't usually take anything for it, 'I just have to sleep it off, it's the only way', although she did resort to pain killers on one occasion 'because my head was so bad'.

Mrs P also described a case in which her husband's illness had not run its typical course. He had developed a chest infection over the week-end and initially refused to see a doctor because 'he thought he'd dose up and shake it off like he's done before'. He eventually did see the doctor and was off work for two weeks with bronchitis. In describing this as 'very unusual for him' Mrs P said:

> (P25) (Mrs P) 'A couple of times he was sick, two different nights. But it still didn't unfortunately make any difference. Now normally, if he is sick it will often clear him of anything if he doesn't feel well, you know, he seems to be fine but he wasn't this time at all.'

The respondents frequently asserted that the remedies they used were successful in resolving the problems for which they were designed even though there was no medical basis for that success. Under the assumption that if A precedes B then A may reasonably be seen to be causing B, the resolution of a problem may be attributed to the remedy that precedes it. Where a theory is available to connect the two, the conclusion that the remedy is an effective cure is reinforced.

Mrs F, for example, invoked a germ theory of disease when explaining the action she or members of her family followed if they had reason to suspect they might get a cold:

> (F29) (Mrs F) 'Before we go to bed we put a little bit of TCP up each nostril, because I think if there's any germs up there, kill them off, mate, before they get any bigger and I will suck a TCP pastille, you know, if there are any germs down there, you know, it's got all night to work on them. As I say, my husband, he'll sniff up TCP if he's been in contact with anyone with a cold or if anybody in the family's got a cold, we say, come on, TCP bottle, you know. Now I wouldn't gargle with it, you see, it's just a case of sniffing a bit up because that's where I feel the germs are probably, you see, up there and down there, that's where they start and if you can knock them out for a bit or weaken them or something with TCP, do so. I hate gargling, I don't think it does you any good quite honestly, you make lovely noises but I feel it probably never gets the water only wiggles about in the space, it never actually

touches anywhere to stay long enough to do anything. I think it's a waste of time.'

As Schutz has pointed out in his analysis of the natural attitude, the commonsense actor has a pragmatic rather than a theoretical orientation to the world. His stock of knowledge at hand and the projects to which it gives rise are only as good as they need to be in bringing about desired ends. Consequently he is not concerned with the preservation of a set of theoretical ideas but will draw on contradictory notions of the way the world works or ideas drawn from conflicting sources in finding solutions, defined as successful according to his own criteria, to the problems with which he is faced.

At the last interview I conducted with Mrs F she was suffering from a 'bad attack' of her allergy. She had been to the doctor for fresh supplies of the drugs she normally used to control the problem and despite 'various ointments and drops and what have you it's not really better'. All the doctor could suggest is that Mrs F went back to see a specialist which, as I have described, she thought was a waste of time. However, there was a further option available to Mrs F:

(F30)   (Mrs F) 'Quite honestly, I'll tell you what I'm going to do, I shall go to the spiritualist's and say what can you do for me because I have been before and I think it's one of those things, they might possibly clear up for me whereas medical science can't.'

In the discussion that followed, Mrs F elaborated on the reasons for her trying spiritual healing:

(F31)   (Mrs F) 'I always used to go quite a lot actually, I used to take my mother to, erm, a dear lady who had, er, a room in Wembley 'cos we had a healer in the family . . .'
     (Int.) 'Yes.'
     (Mrs F) 'you know, my aunt is a spiritual healer and therefore one tends to think, well, you know, there might be something in it. But I wouldn't go to my aunt 'cos we're sort of incompatible, you know, like relations sometimes are. But we did go, my mum and I, to this lady in Wembley and she was a dear and she was a great help to both of us, you know, I sort of had, I first went to her when I had a very bad bout of bronchitis which is something I never get, I think it was sort of a virus bronchitis thing . . .'
     (Int.) 'Mm.'
     (Mrs F) 'and I was singing in a show and, you know, I'd coughed so much my voice had practically gone. Anyway, within two days she had me singing again.'
     (Int.) 'Really?'
     (Mrs F) 'So I went to her just to keep well. Quite honestly, it was

more or less a social occasion, she used to hold a sort of open clinic, you know, everybody sort of walked in, all sat down and had a little chat and you went up to have your treatment, you know, in turn and it was really quite pleasant. As I say, I used to take my mother. She cured me of warts, I also, you know, I used to be susceptible, I had a lot of warts and I had them burned off at the hospital and then I had another batch coming and I said to her, well, I said, look here we go again and she said we'll see if we can do that and she sort of put the fluence on and I sort of forgot about it, she forgot about it and a couple of weeks afterwards I thought my warts have gone. I mean, I know people can . . .'

(Int.) 'Yes.'

(Mrs F) 'warts are funny things they might have gone away on their own anyway but, er, she got rid of those for me. So I think this is what I shall do. I might possibly take my mum as well because she used to get a lot of, seemed to get a lot of relief with her back-aches from this lady we used to go to. So quite honestly, I might as well just go there as go through the hospital pipeline again.'

Spiritual healers may, like other 'fringe' practitioners, be viewed as cranks, frauds, or persons of dubious moral character. They may be condemned for believing in and basing their practices in a system of healing which is ritualistic, magical, and without scientific foundation. This belief in the supernatural may be taken as an indicator of the person's incompetence. Or they may be viewed as individuals who practise a system of medicine which they know is ineffective for financial or other gains. The persons who consult fringe practitioners may, by implication, be similarly viewed. In this extended extract Mrs F elaborates on the value of spiritual healing to justify her decision to seek this type of help. Ultimately, that justification rests upon the fact that spiritual healing is just as likely to produce results as medical science. That Mrs F is able to maintain a belief in both systems of healing requires that problems are conceived of as falling into one of two types depending upon the type of treatment to which they respond. Medical science cannot help as far as her allergy is concerned; consequently it may be a disorder which falls outside the sphere of competence of orthodox medicine as 'one of those things' that spiritual healing 'might possibly clear up'. The contradictions in the systems of thought embodied in the two types of healing are not a problem for Mrs F. From within the natural attitude practical problem solving is of more relevance than matters of theoretical purity.

Mrs F's past experience with spiritual healing has shown her that it can in some circumstances be effective. Following a bad bout of bronchitis in which her voice had practically gone, Mrs F went to a spiritual healer who 'had me singing again within two days'. That this should be recognized as an achievement is emphasized when Mrs F says that bronchitis 'is something I never get'. Mrs F also claims to have been cured of warts which recurred after treatment at the hospital, although she does recognize that alternative formulations are possible, 'warts are funny things they might have gone away on their own anyway', and Mrs F's mother at least seemed to get a lot of relief from back-aches. In addition, the family connection with spiritual healing encourages the view that it may have some validity, and apart from that the healing sessions are of value in themselves as a pleasant social occasion. Mrs F's use of spiritual healing for preventive purposes, 'I went to her just to keep well', was motivated as much by the social as the health gains. In this way Mrs F constructs a definition of spiritual healing such that it may reasonably be seen to be worth a try.

Later in the interview I asked Mrs F why she had suddenly decided to try spiritual healing: she said, 'Well, I haven't had it bad enough for it to worry me and not clear up'. The decision to try a different form of healing was prompted by an episode of her allergy which lasted six weeks in comparison to its normal course of one to two weeks. The failure of her own management routine and the inability of medical science to help meant that her options were limited once it became necessary for something to be done. Spiritual healing was then a last resort.

Unlicensed problem-solvers may be consulted when formal medical care systems fail to provide solutions to problems or they may be consulted in preference to those systems. Pharmacists are partially licensed in the sense that they are able to offer potential solutions to a limited range of problems by means of the proprietary medicines that they sell. This may be extended when they supply preparations normally available only on prescription. The respondents' efforts to manage the disorders they experienced themselves frequently involved the purchase and use of proprietary medicines or asking pharmacists for advice on the best course of action. Mrs S said that she often asked the chemist to make up medicines for her children or asked his advice:

(S47) (Mrs S) 'At Christmas I had this really bad cold and it wasn't just a cold it was a sore throat as well, it was, you know, more like a laryngitis sort of thing but I didn't bother to go to the doctor's, I just got, you know, some cough mixture, I went to, you know, the chemist himself and asked him what was the best thing and he gave me this . . .'

(Int.) 'Do you often do that?'

(Mrs S) 'Oh yes, I often do. The man in the chemist's, you know, I've known him quite a long time, he's nice and friendly, sometimes he'll make up a cough mixture for the youngsters if necessary and if I need any advice sort of thing I'll always ask him. If he can make something up for them he always will. I've always done this 'cos I used to work in a chemist's so I think you know although it wasn't actually behind that particular part we had a lot of people kept asking this sort of thing and I've found they're quite knowledgeable things that they could prescribe, you know, without a doctor then they would do it so, erm, that sort of thing, I've always done since working in there from the age of seventeen.'

Mrs S's biography included experience of working in a chemist's shop and although it 'wasn't actually behind that particular part' it does impart some legitimacy to her actions. She is able to assert that her actions are typical, 'a lot of people kept asking this sort of thing', and reasonable since pharmacists are competent to prescribe, 'I've found they're quite knowledgeable', and willing to do so within the limits of their licence.

Mrs G claimed that she would often attempt to buy things to deal with any problems she or her children might have even though consulting a doctor would allow her to obtain the medicines she would otherwise buy free of charge. Again, Mrs G claimed that this sort of action is typical:

(G40) (Mrs G) 'And yet when you think about it a lot of people do that. In fact, when I bought that cough mixture I was speaking to another woman who's got twins and she'd been buying things for those kids that had this sort of a cold and yet she could get free prescriptions for those children and yet she spent a lot of money, you know, whereas, and the same with me, I went and bought that cough mixture when in fact I could have got it free because I get free National Health prescriptions but I just wouldn't waste his [the doctor's] time.'

Not only does consulting a chemist save a doctor's time, it is deemed a preferable course of action because it requires less effort on the part of the respondent, produces essentially similar outcomes and avoids the potential risks of visiting a busy clinic:

(G41) (Mrs G) 'I know that say, rather than go to the doctor I've bought things, you know, say if it's only cough mixture or something like that. And yet at the same time I've got a National Health Service exemption card which is stupid, isn't it?'
(Int.) 'Mm.'
(Mrs G) 'But I've done it rather than spend time and effort waiting to see the doctor and coming out with a prescription 'cos there's a chemist up here that'll prescribe something for you that's not on the shelf.'
(Int.) 'What that's only supposed to be on prescription?'
(Mrs G) 'Can only be prescribed, yes.'
(Int.) 'Why would you see him rather than go to the doctor?'
(Mrs G) 'I don't know . . . probably the fact that with it being a

clinic it's such a big practice and there's always so many people to see, you go up there with a cough and you come back with German measles, you go up there with a cold and you come back with a sore throat, if you go up for an injection, you know, you come back with somebody else's infections.'

One further option open to individuals faced with disorders of various kinds is to do nothing. Mrs F claimed that doing nothing was her general strategy for coping with signs and symptoms, she ignored them and hoped they would go away. That such rules of procedure may be modified by circumstance is evidenced by some of the data that I have already presented. The time-place contexts in which signs and symptoms are situated may alter their meaning and their implications for action as may the way in which signs and symptoms develop over time. Mrs F's daughter was 'particularly worried' about the heat rash on her face 'because at the moment she's doing photographic modelling' and went to see the doctor. For Mrs F and her family whether or not they were currently involved in an amateur dramatic production formed a context in which health matters were of some concern. When her daughter began to complain of a sore throat just prior to singing the lead in a school production, Mrs F 'dosed her up last night with Lemsip, Vick on the chest, TCP up her nose, cough mixture and what have you, I think come on if you think you're getting a cold 'cos the show's on Tuesday . . .'. When Mrs F told me her husband had a cold I asked if he was doing anything about it:

(F32) (Mrs F) 'Nothing at all. If he were doing a show he would if it were vital for him to be well. But it's not vital, all he's got to do is go to work, he's not bothered.'

Individuals may also assert that they did nothing about problematic experiences affecting themselves or those for whom they are responsible because there was nothing that could be done. When Mrs S's daughter was sick one night Mrs S 'didn't do a thing for her' because 'I really don't think there's much you can do when they're being sick'.

As with all health and illness related actions doing nothing may be legitimated by reference to professional definitions of the situation. Parents may point to such definitions to account for their apparent lack of action with regard to a disorder in one of their children:

(R43) (Mrs R) 'She started getting these pains usually at night and I took her to our previous doctor who said it's probably from cold, ignore it, and it happened quite a few times so I took her back and in fact our previous doctor was away at the time and her locum, I thought it was quite good to get another opinion on it, and her locum said just leave it alone, so you know we tend to ignore it.'

The lower abdominal pains about which Mrs R's daughter complained periodically had received the attention of two doctors who advised Mrs R to ignore it or leave it alone. Neither of the doctors felt it was in the child's interests to pursue the matter by subjecting her to internal examination and the origin of the pain was never definitely diagnosed. Though Mr R said, 'It's an odd one, I've never heard of it before', the doctor's tentative explanation was accepted. Mrs R thought 'it seems to be her age' and hoped she'd grow out of it. In line with the doctor's advice the problem was ignored and as the pain appeared to be lessening nothing further was done about it.

Other data would suggest that professional advice that nothing can be done may stem from the failure to diagnose, that is produce an explanation of, the disorders which may present. While the failure of a lay person to diagnose a problem is not the end of the explanatory line since consulting licensed problem-solvers is always a possibility, where medical science is not able to produce an explanation the individual may have to accept that the source of the trouble is unknown and nothing can be done. Because the cause of Mrs F's allergic response could not be identified her doctors were unable to suggest any definitive treatment, 'here we are fighting in the dark again', and she decided to seek help outside the formal medical care system. When Mrs R's mother's leg suddenly became swollen and painful no diagnosis was forthcoming because of the atypical course that the problem followed.

(R44) (Mrs R) 'She went down to the doctor who said it sounded like all the symptoms of a thrombosis except that it was strange that it had gone so quickly and she was able to walk. The following day she had an appointment for her normal check-up at the hospital and again the doctor said the same thing, sounds like a thrombosis except it disappeared too quickly and really he couldn't suggest any treatment, erm, you know, take it easy for a week and if you're alright carry on as normal and hope it doesn't recur or that the thing the clot, if it was a clot, doesn't come up somewhere else. Erm, but he couldn't do much for her because he didn't know quite what to do. But it appears to be alright so far so we just hope for the best.'

In cases such as these individuals are left to 'accept it', 'learn to live with it' or 'hope for the best'.

Notes

1. For example, Brown and colleagues (1973), studying the role of life events in the onset of depression, solve this problem of reconstruction by themselves imputing meanings to and making judgements about the severity of the life events their respondents describe. These judgements then become the facts on

which the analysis is based. The validity of the procedure is measured by rater agreement: social reality is measured by consensus.

2. Gleeson and Erben (1976) point out that while ethnomethodology has a sophisticated critique of conventional sociology, it cannot account for the dominance of the positivist perspective within the discipline.

3. McHugh (1968) has referred to this as revelation: two events are seen to be connected and the first reinterpreted in terms of what the second signifies.

4. Note that Mrs G is also able to explain the doctor's behaviour and perception of the situation by making assumptions about his interpretation of events and the way these change with accumulating knowledge.

5. Recall that in Chapter 5 Mrs R refused to accept a similar rationale offered by her husband to account for his refusal to see the doctor about his abdominal pain. The acceptability of any rationale may depend on the circumstance in which it is given.

6. See Comarroff (1976). Assumptions such as these concerning doctors' views of patients are not without foundation.

Conclusion

The descriptions offered in the preceding chapters contain a relatively superficial explication of the practices and procedures integral to the cognitive organization of one aspect of experience, that of health and illness. I say superficial since every extract presented could be subject to a more detailed and extensive analysis. Much more is involved in the accounts I have analysed than has been described so far. However, at this stage a wide-ranging, though somewhat elementary, analysis is probably more valuable than an intensive analysis of a more limited set of issues. Chapters 4, 5, and 6 should be seen as mapping out a field of enquiry and providing some guide as to what issues need to be considered when providing a sociological account of illness and its related phenomena.

The common understandings employed by the women I interviewed to make sense of events located within the realm of health, illness, and its associated behaviours consist of knowledge of two types. Firstly, there is knowledge about matters of health and illness *per se*. This may include such things as typifications of the conduct of people who are ill, the typical ways in which given disorders manifest themselves, their typical courses, and the causal connections between events in the world and problems of various kinds. Secondly, they also had at their disposal more general knowledge about such contextual matters as typical experiences of family life, the nature of children and their particular needs and the motives and conduct of particular types of people. All these may be involved in making inferences about and managing problematic experiences. It is by means of the skilful use of these common under-standings that the women were able to display their status as moral persons and competent members. Moreover, by showing that their inferences and actions were reasonable given the resources at their disposal, they were able to defeat potential charges of incompetence and demonstrate adequate performance as mothers and patients. Accounts given in interviews are to be read as such and not as more or less adequate descriptions of some independent reality.

The women I interviewed were alerted to the possibility that something was wrong with themselves or someone they knew by a number of types of event. Prominent among these were what I have termed symptomatological, behavioural, and communicative cues. These cues were seen to be the external manifestations of an underlying disorder or some other explanation was found whereby they were normalized. In some cases these cues were sufficient in themselves to indicate the presence of disorder; more usually, a cue was seen in the context of other cues which preceded or followed to confirm the suspicion that something was wrong. Hence the search of the immediate past or the 'wait and see' strategy employed when one cue did not provide sufficient evidence for a meaning to be located. Not only were given cues elaborated by others in the search for meaning, they were also seen in terms of biographical and time-place contexts so that the individual concerned was construed as unwell and tentative diagnostic labels applied. This contextual elaboration was of some importance where behavioural and communicative cues were concerned since the experiences they document may not be directly available to persons other than the sufferer.

These cues both indicate and are explained by the categories of phenomena to which they are allocated. Where they are seen as pointing to some disorder an explanation of that disorder may, in turn, be sought. Such explanations typically take the form of 'causal theories' whereby some antecedent agent or event is selected from a culturally prescribed range and fitted to the problem in question. Where a causal explanation could not be constructed, the women were often unable to make sense of what had happened. While this may be of limited significance in the case of relatively short-lived experiences, it would seem to have some consequence where the disorder in question is more threatening or long-term. The cultural resources available to make sense of these experiences do occasionally fail, leaving an individual bewildered or confused. In a secular industrial society witchcraft and God's will can no longer be employed to explain the otherwise inexplicable. As a result, the assumption of a stable, orderly world in which things happen for a reason is sometimes challenged.

The accounts on which these analyses are based demonstrate something of the emergent and transient character of social reality. The objects attended to by man in everyday life are fluid and ambiguous. They change over time as new evidence is accumulated and events subject to retrospective reinterpretation. This accounts for much of the tentative character of lay theorizing and such general interpretive strategies as waiting for future developments under the assumption that these will allow a more certain allocation of experience to socially available categories. That these objects are ambiguous and commonsense theorizing about them is tentative is evidenced by the tendency for the respondents to preface many of their remarks with statements such as 'I don't really know but . . .' and the like. Such ambiguity may arise because the cultural resources available at any given point in time are not adequate for the interpretive task at hand or because those resources offer alternative characterizations or explanations of experienced events. Consequently, this means that any characterization or explanation that is offered may be shown to be inadequate in the light of subsequent experience.[1]

However, although events and experiences are essentially ambiguous, they are not necessarily perceived as such by the participants in everyday life. They are frequently able to fit a description to a scene and make sense of what is going on in much the same way as they are able to understand what people say, even though utterances can always be taken to mean more than one thing.[2] This highlights the extent to which social order is an accomplishment, 'a construction of and constituted by the activities of people's minds' (Wootton 1975:96).

In Chapter 5 I described the way in which ideas not too dissimilar from those outlined by Parsons in his discussion of the sick role were used as an interpretive device in talk about health and illness. They were used both in the construction of definitions and as prescriptions for action. I argued that illness is one explanation of patterns of action I called illness-relevant behaviours. Actions such staying in bed, not going to work, going to see the doctor are typical of people who are ill. Consequently, anyone who undertakes these actions may be allocated to that category and anyone who claims to be ill can be expected to pursue action of this kind. Failure to do so may result in the definition 'ill' being denied unless acceptable reasons can be found to justify that failure.

Because actions of this kind may be motivated by a desire for the benefits they involve, a definition of illness assumes and may only be applied where they are seen to be the unavoidable outcome of some underlying disorder or the subjective experiences to which it gives rise. Where no underlying disorder can be identified, or where its presence is ambiguous, then alternative formulations such as malingering may be considered. This is particularly the case with mental illness and other problems involving subjective states where the disorder has no externally available manifestations other than the claims or behaviour of the sufferer.

Because imputations of illness locate the origins of conduct in an underlying biological disorder the individual so labelled is absolved of responsibility for his actions. Consequently, illness is essentially a moral category; it always involves judgements about the extent to which an individual has personal control over his actions. Moreover, illness and deviance are mutually exclusive, alternative explanations of given states of affairs, so that it is not possible to talk of illness as deviance *per se*. Imputations of deviance explain behaviour in terms of socially appropriate motives and goals while definitions of illness do not. Since the labelling of someone as ill necessarily involves such judgements it is a social phenomenon quite distinct from the biological abnormalities with which it is sometimes associated.

While interview talk may lend itself to an investigation of the interpretive procedures involved in the construction of definitions of illness and the recognition and explanation of disorder, it is subject to certain limitations when used for the study of illness behaviour. For if accounts of actions undertaken to manage problematic experiences are interpretive rather than literal descriptions, then it is not possible to use these accounts to say what meanings were imputed to events in the past or to show how they gave rise to the action in question. They can only be used to show how actions are constituted as rational acts. Since it is not possible to get inside someone else's head it may not be possible to show a direct connection between meaning and action no matter what kind of data is collected. Consequently, the proposition that people act towards objects on the basis of the meanings those objects hold for them has the status of a philosophical assumption that is no more open to verification than the idea that social reality is a cognitive construct. What this means is that while an appreciation of social action is possible the production of a distinctly sociological explanation of that action is somewhat problematic.

That the women I interviewed took for granted the reasonableness of their actions was inherent in much of what they said. They depicted their doctors as busy men who should not be bothered with trivial disorders that anyone might be expected to treat themselves. They claimed that they only consulted the doctor with problems that were significant or warranted special attention, since these could have indicated a serious disorder or fallen outside a lay person's competence. Moreover, they presented themselves as competent to judge when such professional attention was necessary. Only children were exempt from this general rule and they were frequently taken to see the doctor 'just to be on the safe side'. Consequently, any challenge to this assumption of competence and rationality often brought forth a complaint on their part.

In explaining their own actions or the actions of others, the respondents often made reference to the way in which the object of those actions was interpreted. When called to account for any delay in visiting the doctor they pointed to the triviality of the problem in question or the fact that it had not been seen as a problem at all. These interpretations were justified on the grounds that they were reasonable given the facts that were available at the time. Subsequent visits to the doctor were presented as following a reinterpretation of the problem brought about by the advent of a critical incident. These critical incidents figure in cases where alternative meanings could have been applied to the problem being reviewed. They were absent from those cases in which the only available meaning to make sense of the problem indicated a potentially serious disorder. Here, going to see the doctor was motivated by a desire to have the tentative diagnosis confirmed or denied. Because problematic experiences were often ambiguous and could not always be un-equivocally deemed to require medical attention, a 'wait and see' strategy was adopted, and decisions were suspended pending future developments. In this respect the respondents made use of assumptions about the typical course of given types of problems in order to assign meaning and to plan action.

Two types of external constraint were presented as being relevant to the decision to seek medical attention. First, constraints on resources such as time were imposed by the responsibilities associated with the statuses the women occupied. As wives and mothers they were expected to put the interests of family first so gave preference to their household duties rather than their own needs for medical attention. Second, they identified a number of interactional and organizational barriers which they claimed had an influence on their help-seeking behaviour. Some negotiation was required to circumvent these barriers so that access could be gained to a consultation and their self-defined needs fulfilled. These barriers not only constitute the rationale for not seeing the doctor, they provide the grounds on which criticisms of · medical care may be constructed. However, they are only good reasons for acting in particular ways, and cause for complaint, if recognized as such by reference to a stock of knowledge which includes typifications of patients' experiences with medical practice. That they are typical is to be read from the respondents' assertions that 'they happen to the majority'. One method of coping with these barriers is not to attempt to circumvent them but to seek alternative methods of managing problems and other sources of help.

I have indicated that there are two aspects of the construction of meanings that may be analysed sociologically, the cognitive and interactional dimensions. The former refers to the organization and interpretation of events and the production via language of a recognizable social order. The latter refers to the location of meaning construction within interpersonal activity. The meanings that individuals construct are frequently, if not always, influenced by those with whom they interact. This influence may be direct, as in various forms of negotiation where meanings are overtly problematic. Or it may be indirect, where meanings are not in dispute but constrained by the fact that they must be adequate for the others involved in the situations in which they are used. Meanings always involve joint effort; cognitive processes must be utilized both in their production by one party and in their interpreta-tion by another. Here, I am primarily concerned with the former, since the latter would be confined to an examination of the pro-duction and negotiation of meanings within the context of a research interview.[3] While I assume that those meanings are a product of inter-viewer-interviewee interaction, the cognitive processes involved are not confined to that particular context but may well be employed in others.

The foregoing analysis would suggest that doctors' complaints about the number of trivial conditions that present in general practice stem from their tendency to view patients and their problems from a perspective in which judgements about the clinical significance of problematic experiences provide for judgements about the appropriateness of help-seeking behaviour. The data in Chapters 4, 5, and 6 contain a different model of rationality and a different way of viewing such behaviour. Significance and rationality are not labels that can be legitimately employed without specification of an interpretive context. Consequently, what are irrational or inappropriate consultations from one position may not be so from another; that is, if they are seen in terms of the knowledge, resources, interests, and responsibilities of the individual concerned. By employing devices of this kind the respondents were able to provide for the reasonableness of the way in which they interpreted the world and what they subsequently did. By employing a similar set of devices, those involved in the delivery of medical care may be better able to understand the conduct of those with whom they come into contact.

By conveying something of the complexity of social life in general and social interaction in particular, the analysis may also stimulate an awareness of how statements and actions on the part of those who provide or control access to medical care can often be interpreted as challenges to the patient's status as a competent member and responsible person. This not only creates covert conflict, it also exacerbates the dilemma that individuals face in their attempts to make sense of and cope with their problems. Acting according to their own definitions of what is necessary to solve their problems, whether these are practical or cognitive, may be inconsistent with professional ideas of what constitutes a good patient. Children are a particular problem in this respect since they are not always able to provide detailed descriptions of their subjective experiences and because it is assumed that symptoms of any kind may be indicative of relatively serious disorders. Seeking professional advice not only provides a solution to these diagnostic uncertainties, it also has a symbolic value by indicating parental concern and proper care of the child. It is because such behaviour can be faulted and labelled as the action of an over-protective or fussy parent that patients may develop strategies for defusing or circumventing these interpretive differences. However, an understanding of help-seeking behaviour and its potential for avoiding these kinds of interactional difficulties is only likely to be of importance if medicine is taken to be a body of knowledge applied to people's problems rather than to their biological abnormalities.

Notes

1. This must call into question the status of responses to questionnaires designed to measure the prevalence of signs and symptoms. These responses are not literal descriptions of objective events but retrospective reconstructions which are liable to change over time.
2. The most striking illustrations of this are the experiments by Garfinkel (1967) and McHugh (1968) where subjects were able to make sense of random responses to their utterances.
3. These meanings are negotiated in so far as the questions asked by the interviewer provide the respondents with frames of reference for organizing their experience. It should be noted that these questions presuppose the topics that it is the analytic task to describe. The respondents' descriptions and the questions that generate them both presume commonsense knowledge of social structures. More overt negotiation of meanings occurs where the interviewer is called upon to offer formulations of the events the respondents have encountered.

References

Atkinson, J.M. (1978) *Discovering Suicide: The Social Organisation of Sudden Death*. London: Macmillan Press.

Beales, G. (1976) Practical Sociological Reasoning and the Making of Social Relationships among Health Centre Participants. In M. Stacey (ed.) *The Sociology of the NHS*. Sociological Review Monograph No. 22.

Becker, H. (1963) *The Outsiders*. New York: Free Press.

Bloor, M. and Horobin, G. (1975) Conflict and Conflict Resolution in Doctor-Patient Interactions. In C. Cóx and A. Meade (eds) *A Sociology of Medical Practice*. London: Collier-Macmillan.

Blumer, H. (1966) Sociological Implications of the Thought of George Herbert Mead. *American Journal of Sociology* **71**: 535–44.

—— (1969) *Symbolic Interactionism*. Englewood Cliffs, NJ: Prentice-Hall.

Bott, E. (1971) *The Family and Social Network*. London: Tavistock Publications.

Box, S. (1971) *Deviance, Reality and Society*. London: Holt, Reinhardt and Winston.

Brown, G., Sklair, F., Harris, T., and Birley, J. (1973) Life Events and Psychiatric Disorder: Some Methodological Issues. *Psychological Medicine* **3**: 74–87.

Burton, L. (1975) *The Family Life of Sick Children*. London: Routledge and Kegan Paul.

Butler, J. (1970) Illness and the Sick Role: an Evaluation in Three Communities. *British Journal of Sociology* **21**: 241–61.

Cartwright, A. (1967) *Patients and their Doctors*. London: Routledge and Kegan Paul.

Cicourel, A. (1964) *Method and Measurement in Sociology*. New York: Free Press.

—— (1968) *The Social Organisation of Juvenile Justice*. New York: Wiley and Sons.

—— (1973) *Cognitive Sociology*. Harmondsworth, Middlesex: Penguin.

Comarroff, J. (1976) Communicating Information about Non-Fatal Illness: the Strategies of a Group of General Practitioners. *Sociological Review* **24**: 269–90.

Coulter, J. (1974) *Approaches to Insanity*. London: Martin Robertson.

Cowie, B. (1976) The Cardiac Patient's Perception of His Heart Attack. *Social Science and Medicine* **10**: 87–96.

Cunningham, D. (1978) *Stigma and Social Isolation: A Study of MS Patients.* Health Services Research Unit, University of Kent.

Davis, A. and Strong, P. (1976) Aren't Children Wonderful? A Study of the Allocation of Identity in Developmental Assessment. In M. Stacey (ed.) *The Sociology of the NHS.* Sociological Review Monograph No. 22.

Davis, F. (1963) *Passage Through Crisis: Polio Victims and their Families.* Indianapolis: Bobbs-Merrill.

Dingwall, R. (1976) *Aspects of Illness.* London: Martin Robertson.

Douglas, J. (1971a) *American Social Order.* New York: Free Press.

—— (1971b) *Understanding Everyday Life.* London: Routledge and Kegan Paul.

—— (1972) (ed.) *Research on Deviance.* New York: Random House.

Engel, G. (1960) A Unified Concept of Health and Illness. *Perspectives in Biology and Medicine* **3**: 459–85.

Fabrega, H. (1972) The Study of Disease in Relation to Culture. *Behavioural Science* **17**: 183–203.

Fabrega, H. and Manning, P. (1972) Disease, Illness and Deviant Careers. In P. Scott and J. Douglas (eds) *Theoretical Perspectives on Deviance.* New York: Basic Books.

Fay, B. (1973) *Social Theory and Political Practice.* London: George Allen and Unwin.

Field, D. (1976) The Social Definition of Illness. In D. Tuckett (ed.) *An Introduction to Medical Sociology.* London: Tavistock Publications.

Filmer, P., Phillipson, M., Silverman, D., and Walsh, D. (1972) *New Directions in Sociological Theory.* New York: Cromwell Collier-Macmillan.

Freidson, E. (1970a) *Professional Dominance: the Social Structure of Medical Care.* New York: Atherton Press.

—— (1970b) *The Profession of Medicine.* New York: Dodds Mead and Co.

Garfinkel, H. (1956) Conditions of Successful Degradation Ceremonies. *American Journal of Sociology* **61**: 420–4.

—— (1967) *Studies in Ethnomethodology.* Englewood Cliffs, NJ: Prentice-Hall.

Gibbs, J.P. (1966) Conceptions of Deviant Behaviour: the Old and the New. *Pacific Sociological Review* **9**: 9–14.

Giddens, A. (1976) *New Rules of Sociological Method.* London: Hutchinson.

Gleeson, D. and Erben, M. (1976) Meaning in Context: Notes towards a Critique of Ethnomethodology. *British Journal of Sociology* **27**: 474–83.

Goffman, E. (1968) *Asylums.* Harmondsworth, Middlesex: Penguin.

Gordon, G. (1966) *Role Theory and Illness.* New Haven, Conn.: College and University Press.

Gough, H. (1977) Doctors' Estimates of the Percentage of Patients who do not require Medical Treatment. *Medical Education* **II**: 380–4.

Kasl, V. and Cobb, S. (1966) Health Behaviour, Illness Behaviour, and Sick Role Behaviour. *Archives of Environmental Health* **12**: 246–66.

Kassebaum, G. and Baumann, B. (1965) Dimensions of the Sick Role in Chronic Illness. *Journal of Health and Social Behaviour* **16**: 16–27.

Kosa, J. and Robertson, S. (1969) Social Aspects of Health and Illness. In J. Kosa, *et al.* (eds) *Poverty and Health: A Sociological Analysis.* Cambridge, Mass.: Harvard University Press.

Lemert, E. (1967) *Human Deviance, Social Problems and Social Control.* Englewood Cliffs, NJ: Prentice-Hall.

—— (1971) *Social Pathology.* New York: McGraw-Hill.

Linsky, A.A. (1970) Who Shall be Excluded: The Influence of Personal Attributes in Community Reaction to the Mentally Ill. *Social Psychiatry* **5**: 166–71.

Litman, T. (1974) The Family as a Basic Unit in Health and Medical Care. *Social Science and Medicine* **8**: 495–519.

Locker, D. (1979) *Symptoms and Illness: The Cognitive Organization of Disorder.* Thesis submitted for the degree of PhD. University of Kent.

McCall, G. and Simmons, J. (1969) *Issues in Participant Observation.* Reading, Mass.: Addison Wesley.

McHugh, P. (1968) *Defining the Situation: The Organisation of Meaning in Social Interaction.* Indianapolis: Bobbs-Merrill.

—— (1970) A Commonsense Conception of Deviance. In J. Douglas (ed.) *Deviance and Respectability.* New York: Basic Books.

Mankoff, M. (1971) Societal Reaction and Career Deviance: A Critical Analysis. *Sociological Quarterly* **12**: 204–18.

Manning, P. (1971) Talking and Becoming: A View of Organisational Socialisation. In J. Douglas (ed.) *Understanding Everyday Life.* London: Routledge and Kegan Paul.

Mechanic, D. (1962) The Concept of Illness Behaviour. *Journal of Chronic Disease* **15**: 189–94.

—— (1974) *Politics, Medicine and Social Science.* New York: Wiley Interscience.

Moore, M. (1974) Demonstrating the Rationality of an Occupation. *Sociology* **8**: 110–21.

Morgan, D. (1975) Explaining Mental Illness. *Archives of European Sociology* **16**: 268–79.

Parsons, T. (1951) *The Social System.* Glencoe, Ill.: Free Press.

—— (1958) Definitions of Health and Illness in the Light of the American Social Structure. In E. Jaco (ed.) *Patients, Physicians and Illness.* Glencoe, Ill.: Free Press.

Pearson, G. (1975) *The Deviant Imagination.* London: Macmillan Press.

Pflanz, M. and Rhode, J. (1970) Illness: Deviant Behaviour or Conformity? *Social Science and Medicine* **4**: 645–53.

Pollner, M. (1974) Sociological and Commonsense Models of the

Labelling Process. In R. Turner (ed.) *Ethnomethodology*. Harmonds-worth, Middlesex: Penguin.

Puccetti, R. (1968) *Persons: A Study of Possible Moral Agents in the Universe*. London: Macmillan Press.

Robinson, D. (1971) *The Process of Becoming Ill*. London: Routledge and Kegan Paul.

Schutz, A. (1962) *Collected Papers Vol I: The Problem of Social Reality*. The Hague: Martinuss Nijhof.

Sedgwick, P. (1972) *Mental Illness is Illness*. Paper presented to National Deviancy Conference, York.

Smart, B. (1976) *Sociology, Phenomenology and Marxian Analysis*. London: Routledge and Kegan Paul.

Smith, D. (1972) K is Mentally Ill: The Anatomy of a Factual Account. *Sociology* **12**: 23–53.

Stacey, M. (1976) *Concepts of Health and Illness: A Working Paper on the Concepts and their Relevance for Research*. Social Science Research Council.

Stimson, G. and Webb, B. (1976) People's Accounts of Medical Encounters. In D. Robinson and M. Wadsworth (eds), *Studies in Everyday Medical Life*. London: Martin Robertson.

Suchman, A.E. (1965) Stages of Illness and Medical Care. *Journal of Health and Social Behaviour* **6**: 114–28.

Sudnow, D. (1973) Normal Crimes. In E. Rubington and M. Weinberg (eds) *Deviance: The Interactionist Perspective*. New York: Macmillan.

Szasz, T. (1961) *The Myth of Mental Illness*. New York: Harper and Row.

Taylor, I., Walton, P., and Young, J. (1973) *The New Criminology*. London: Routledge and Kegan Paul.

Turner, R. (1968) The Self Conception in Social Interaction. In K. Gergen and J. Gordon (eds) *The Self in Social Interaction*. New York: Wiley and Sons.

—— (1971) Words, Utterances and Activities. In J. Douglas (ed.) *Understanding Everyday Life*. London: Routledge and Kegan Paul.

Voysey, M. (1975) *A Constant Burden: The Reconstitution of Family Life*. London: Routledge and Kegan Paul.

Wagner, H.R. (ed.) (1970) *Alfred Schutz on Phenomenology and Social Relations*. Chicago: University of Chicago Press.

Whatmore, R., Duward, L., and Kushlik, A. (1974) The Use of the Behaviour Modification Model in Attempting to Derive a Measure of the Quality of Residential Care – Some Methodological Problems. *Behaviour Research and Therapy* **13**: 227–36.

Wilson, T. (1971) Normative and Interpretive Paradigms in Sociology. In J. Douglas (ed.) *Understanding Everyday Life*. London: Routledge and Kegan Paul.

Wing, J. and Brown, G. (1970) *Institutionalism and Schizophrenia*. Cambridge: Cambridge University Press.

Wootton, A. (1975) *Dilemmas of Discourse: Controversies in the Sociological Interpretation of Language.* London: George Allen and Unwin.

Yarrow, M., Schwartz, C., Murphy, H., and Deasy, L. (1973) The Psychological Meaning of Mental Illness in the Family. In Rubington, E. and Weinberg, M. (eds) *Deviance: The Interactionist Perspective.* New York: Macmillan.

Zimmerman, D. and Weider, D. (1971) Ethnomethodology and the Problem of Order. In J. Douglas (ed.) *Understanding Everyday Life.* London: Routledge and Kegan Paul.

Zola, I. (1973) Pathways to the Doctor: From Person to Patient. *Social Science and Medicine* **7**: 677–88.

Subject index

Name index

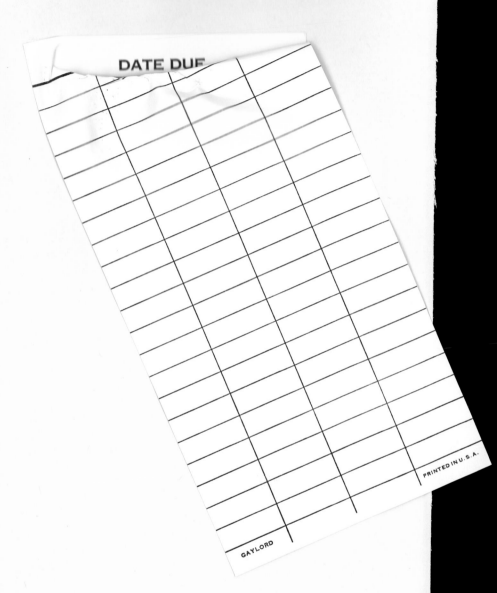

DATE DUE

GAYLORD   PRINTED IN U.S.A.